About the Authors

INGRID ROSE Ph.D.

Ingrid has been in private practice for more than 30 years working with a large range of presentations, as well as being a clinical supervisor and group facilitator. She has taught at college level, and offers training and workshops in many countries of the world. Ingrid also has a long history of yoga and meditation practice, and a strong interest in shamanism.

KAY RYAN MHSc; Dipl.PW, RPBANZ; MIOPOP.

Kay is a registered psychotherapist in private practice and a founding member of Process Oriented Psychology in New Zealand. She has been on the faculty of Australian/New Zealand Process Oriented Psychology She has a long term interest in how dreams and dream-like experiences assist us through life's transitions. She is the Spiritual Support Coordinator at a local hospice where she assists patients, families, staff and volunteers in care of the dying.

Ingrid Rose and Kay Ryan

DOORWAYS INTO DYING: INNOVATIVE TEACHINGS FOR END OF LIFE

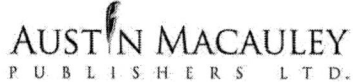

AUSTIN MACAULEY
PUBLISHERS LTD.

A CIP catalogue record for this title is available from the British Library.

ISBN 9781786126344 (Paperback)
ISBN 9781786126351 (Hardback)
ISBN 9781786126368 (E-Book)

www.austinmacauley.com

First Published (2016)
Austin Macauley Publishers Ltd.
25 Canada Square
Canary Wharf
London
E14 5LQ

Acknowledgments

Much gratitude and appreciation go to Arnold and Amy Mindell, our teachers, who have been pioneers in this field, and who have demonstrated that it is possible to make contact with individuals who appear to be non-responsive, and whom family members, hospital staff, and caregivers deem unreachable. Their unique skills, creativity and openness have provided deep teaching for us, modelling a way to engage meaningfully with process in all the ways in which it manifests.

We are appreciative of participants in our workshops and students of our certificate programs from whom we have learned so much. Thank you also to the dedicated hospice and aged care facility staff who apply the methods we teach and continue to inspire us with their own wisdom and experience

In this book we have used examples from our work with patients and families. We are deeply grateful for their generosity in permitting us to share their stories.

Kay particularly acknowledges the learning gained from being alongside her late husband Mike as she participated in his dying process.

We also wish to acknowledge each other for the unique contribution we have each made to our work together, and for our impressive teamwork.

Contents

PART I

Introduction

"I am not afraid of death just the process of getting there" and "I don't know how to die" are phases often heard from patients nearing the end of their lives. They reveal a growing interest, even curiosity about the experience of dying and how to go through it. Historically, ideas and practices around death and dying have changed along with the evolution of society. From earliest times dying was a community event. People died at home surrounded by family and community. Today, with medicalization of dying, we are more likely to place ourselves in the hands of professionals, doctors, nurses, counsellors, social workers, and chaplains, who take responsibility for managing the ways in which a person dies. We know that with the availability of more aggressive treatments and medications, many of us will reach an advanced age, and so we are living longer with the prospect of dying stretched out ahead of us. If we so choose, we have time to reflect and plan our dying while still living a relatively full life. Of course advances in the study of aging and medicine also mean that we can push death even further away and focus on living.

The well-managed, and timely death has become a primary focus, at least in the West. One of the difficulties and challenges with this kind of management of death and dying is that there are dimensions of the dying process that do not respond to a linear and programmed approach. These include the unexpected and often spontaneous expressions in sound and movement, mysterious visions, surprising relationship events and spiritual insights. It has also been found that when the dying process is somewhat chaotic or untimely, the patient may feel guilt and shame and think they are doing something wrong.

Many professionals and family members caring for the dying are aware that the biomedical model does not go far enough to address non-physical aspects of the dying process. We may get caught in the dilemma of whether to use medication, or not, not knowing what else to do for something that appears to be meaningful to the patient. In many cases the importance of experiences such as visions, confusion, delirium, dementia, transpersonal dreams, conflicts, altered states of consciousness, and spiritual phenomena are minimised or explained as being part of the dying brain. We don't quite know how to address these phenomena and so they tend to get pushed aside and often ignored.

We are challenged to find another approach to dying, one that views all experiences as holding potential meaning for the dying person.

People do not operate simply as machines that can break down and be repaired: people are full of potential growth in all states of consciousness even up to and perhaps beyond the moment of death.[1]

How do we address the mysterious, unknown, sentient experiences of the dying when little is known about what is happening internally for the patient? Is there a way we can accompany and assist the dying based on the experiences they present? How can we approach death and dying in a way that values all experience as holding potential meaning for the patient even when those experiences are disturbing?

In this book we hope to address these questions through the introduction of theoretical concepts, case studies and examples, as well as exercises for the reader to practise. Part I introduces theory and gives techniques and tools useful in practise. Part II is in the form of a manual and provides exercises for individual inner work, interventions with clients, and also with family members and attending staff. We hope this format will be useful to you.

We have laid out the chapters in a progression that we believe will facilitate a growing understanding as the reader advances through them.

Chapter 1 addresses the transformative aspect of the dying process as personal identity falls away. Chapter 2 explores ideas related to the structure of the dying process and offers techniques for joining and following the patient in their experience. Chapter 3 looks at the continuum of states of consciousness that is often present for the patient, and provides tips and tools for

---

[1] Mindell, A. (2008) *Coma: The Dreambody near Death*

understanding and supporting the patient in their unique process. Chapter 4 provides an alternative way of viewing and working with delirium and dementia. Chapter 5 explains the use of metaphor and dreams in working with the dying and looks at spiritual dimensions and how to support the patient on their mythical path. In chapter 6 we explore the experience of pain and what may lie within it that is useful for the patient. Chapter 7 addresses the larger field surrounding the patient and provides useful information about how to support and enliven relationships, the family and the systemic context in which the patient finds him/herself. In chapter 8, we summarize our ideas and suggest ways in which the reader may begin to apply new skills and awareness. In Part II of the book, we provide the reader with a series of exercises to practice in order to enhance skills that are useful in accompanying the dying and those around them.

The authors, Ingrid Rose and Kay Ryan are currently involved in practising and teaching the skills and techniques described in this book. Over the past eight years they have offered training courses in New Zealand and Australia to doctors, nurses, psychologists, counsellors, social workers, chaplains, carers, family members, as well as those with terminal illness. This manual is a collection of the tools, skills and techniques both learned and taught by them over the years.

Personal Introduction by Ingrid Rose

As I walk into the private room in the hospital, the first thing that catches my eye is a huge mound of a person lying in the hospital bed. She has been in a deep coma for 5 years, kept alive by the tubes and machines connected to her body. I am shadowing my teachers and mentors who have spent years exploring how to engage and make contact with patients in deep out-of-ordinary, vegetative or comatose states. They have invited me along in order to learn more about the kind of work they are doing in this arena.

Sitting next to the woman in the bed is her husband. He is the person who has accompanied her over the years. He insists that she is present and knows what happens around her. As he strokes her hand and talks to her, yet again reassuring her that she is okay and things will be alright, tears leak out from her closed eyelids and slowly trickle down her cheeks. I imagine being in her situation and what it must be like to lay there for 5 years, unable to communicate, unable to reach out and touch, to have a preference met. And yet … it seems there are feelings inside, and in the moment, the means of expression of these is through tears.

We verbally acknowledge her tears, hold her hand, at the same time scanning her huge form, face, arms, and legs, in order to notice whether there are other signs of expression. Generally, people in deep non-verbal states will show small movements such as flickers of the eyebrows, twitches of the lips, repetitive movements of the fingers, hands or feet. When these movements repeat themselves over extended periods of time, it may become possible to use one of these signals in the creation of a binary communication system with the patient. We have then created a bridge between the patient's world and the outer situation, by means of which patients can participate in their treatment and make life/death decisions (see Chapter 2).

I continued to visit the above patient for some weeks before she was moved to another facility where my visits were no longer permitted. I mention her here, as she was the inspiration that led to my becoming more engaged in *Comawork*[2], which later extended to my broader involvement in palliative care and my work with those near-death and in the dying process. I feel very fortunate to have been invited by families and caregivers into these most intimate moments in a person's life and death, and will treasure forever the jewels of wisdom gained through accompanying the dying on their journeys.

Much gratitude and appreciation go to Arnold and Amy Mindell, my teachers, who have been pioneers in this field, and who have demonstrated that it is possible to make contact with individuals who appear to be incommunicado, and whom family members, hospital staff, and caregivers deem unreachable. Their unique skills, creativity and openness have provided deep teaching for me, and have modelled a way to engage meaningfully with the process that unfolds before our eyes, but in the face of which, many of us feel so helpless.

My colleague, Kay Ryan, and I have been giving training seminars together in New Zealand since 2006. I'm indebted to Kay for her ongoing dedication and

---

[2] Mindell, A. (2008). *Coma: The Dreambody near Death*

steadfastness in taking our work further, as well as her ability to be playful and humorous in the toughest moments. This book is the result of the many techniques and ideas that we have imparted to seminar participants who have come to study with us. I see myself as both a teacher and learner in this field, feeling enriched in both my knowledge and practice by the depth, insight and skill of those who have come to learn and share with us. And, of course, the greatest teachers for me have been the clients/patients with whom I have shared many moments of those far-out states; moments of fear, loss, joy, confusion, resistance, love and other-worldliness; the whole gamut of human experience found within the passages of dying and death.

Ingrid Rose has practiced as a psychologist and group facilitator since 1984. Originally South African, she moved to Australia where she lived for some years before relocating to Oregon, USA, to further her practice of Process-oriented Psychology. She is now a faculty member of the Process Work Institute. Ingrid is in private practice and gives trainings and workshops internationally.

Personal Introduction by Kay Ryan

For many years I have been drawn to study what happens to us as we go through major transitions in life such as birth, marriage, mid-life and death. I have observed the many ways we make meaning of what is happening at these times. In recent years I have applied this study, both personally and professionally, to work with the dying. As many of you will know, experiencing the reality of a loved one dying and being responsible for their care, is perhaps one of the most difficult tasks we may ever undertake. We can be unprepared for it. Ten years ago my husband Mike was diagnosed with prostate cancer. The cancer was too advanced for an operation. He was prescribed radiation therapy and medication for pain. Over the years Mike gradually lost his independence, became depressed with increasing pain and inability to do the things he loved. He also experienced small strokes or TIAs, which meant he was becoming more forgetful.

Twelve months before he died he went into private hospital care where I continued watching over and supporting him until his death. We had some difficult and interesting times together. For example, one day when I was feeling exhausted from working full-time, and seeing Mike in the evenings, I walked into his room. He had recently asked for his bed to be turned to face the window so he could see the trees and rolling hills. On that day he was looking out the window, his eyes unfocused, seeing something I could not see. I did not want to disturb him but sat quietly by his bed encouraging him to keep looking at what he was seeing. After a short time, he said: "The boat is coming into the harbour". He then realised I was there and greeted me brightly – "Oh hello darling!" In that brief interaction I knew I would be fine. I loved his dreaming. I felt excited, relieved and sad at how things were moving. Over the next days we followed the movement of the "boat" as it came into the wharf and got ready to sail, as a way to inform us about his dying process.

To be able to assist and support Mike's dying through bringing in my own feelings and dreaming, following his dreams, negotiating with staff, assisting him to find meaning in his delirium and confused states, singing, laughing, and crying together, connecting to his Christian beliefs, and witnessing how he prepared himself to let go of what he knew, was transforming for both of us. I have had many similar experiences with patients and their families in my hospice work.

I have been greatly influenced by the innovative work of Arny and Amy Mindell. I am deeply grateful for their inspiration and wisdom. Their work communicating with people in altered states of consciousness has been particularly useful in working with the dying. Over the past eight years I have been fortunate to teach and facilitate groups with my colleague Ingrid Rose. Together we have applied process-oriented ideas and skills to Palliative Care. Ingrid's insight, compassion, wisdom, depth of knowledge and experience, have inspired and encouraged me.

There is still much to learn about dying. My hope is that you will find that the ideas and techniques in this book will expand your learning and provide you with a way to support and unfold the many extraordinary, creative experiences that can emerge through the dying process and beyond. May it create a pathway for your own dying and enrich your living.

Kay Ryan is a registered Psychotherapist, supervisor and facilitator with over 30 years' experience working in private practice and within various organizations. She has worked in Palliative Care for eight years applying Process-oriented Psychology to her work with patients, families, staff, and volunteers. She has presented papers at several Palliative Care Conferences in Australia and New Zealand. Kay is currently working at a local hospice as a Spiritual Care Coordinator, providing resources and training in end of life care.

Chapter 1

Death – The Transformative Process

When I let go of what I am,
I become what I might be.

- Lao Tse

Throughout life we go through many transformations and little "deaths". Life brings its lessons as we move through its various stages or passages, calling on us to shed parts of ourselves just as a snake sheds its skin. In order to meet new challenges, adapt to a changing world, and grow in self-awareness, new aspects of ourselves emerge as old ones disappear or transform.

The process of psychological development traces the various stages inherent in existence as one moves through a natural progression of renewing the personality on the path of striving for wholeness[3]. In some of us, this may be a conscious attempt to maintain

---

[3] von Franz (1984) *On Dreams and Death*

awareness while meeting the various aspects of ourselves that we encounter at different stages of life. We may work on ourselves, in order to guide the unfolding of new insight as we transform parts from the old into the new. For others of us, there is no conscious awareness of what is transpiring psychologically or spiritually. The process becomes more of an organic path that carries us through the passages of change without much conscious recognition of what is unfolding for us intra-psychically.

At some point, we all find ourselves entering the dying process in which we face a culmination of the path we have been on during a lifetime; a path that has brought moments or periods of transformation, often accompanied by challenge, joy or loss. It is during the dying process that the call to transform is speeded up and we are brought face-to-face with our everyday dying reality, shocking some of us into awakening to the call, or sending others of us into a place of resistance and denial. Those who have held the transformative process in their awareness either through self-exploration or a spiritual practice in their lives, may be more prepared for this dying experience and thus more able to embrace it with openness, harnessing the richness and deep wisdom it may bring. Those who have not, can feel more challenged in letting go as death nears and may struggle or resist, leading to more fear and emotional pain (see example on page 8). In either case, it is rare to find a person effortlessly engaging with death and feeling at home with it.

The experience of dying, although unique to each individual, reveals recognizable patterns or phases. These phases do not occur in a linear progression, but may appear at different times during the death process.

• Denial, anger, the sense of being in a dream or the experience not being real.

• With the prospect of death, we may feel a push to fulfill our lives, to complete unfinished tasks that hold meaning for us. Questions may emerge such as, "Has my life had meaning"? "What is there I still need to do"?

• We encounter experiences of altered states of consciousness such as memory loss, fatigue, delirium, agitation, depression, ecstasy and joy.

• We are faced with the threat of extreme states of consciousness such as coma, paralyzing terror, grief, etc.

• We discover ways to make spiritual connections through visions or out of body experiences.

In any event, it often happens with those who are seriously ill or nearing death that there appear to be states of withdrawal, absent-mindedness, or somewhat altered/irrational cognitive patterns that seem to be inexplicable to the observer. These may go on for some time and the closer to death one gets, the more this may become the "usual" way of expressing or being. Even though we may not be able to make sense out of these patterns, we can still support the ill or dying patient, or family member, to believe in and trust the experience. We can guide them to follow the less known experiences in the way they appear in their inner worlds, believing that these kinds of experiences take the individual further along their path, bringing meaning for them in their process. In joining patients in this space, we can assist in taking the process further.

The Big Ship

Arnold Mindell[4] provides a wonderful example of interacting with an 80-year-old patient, close to death, who was disturbing other patients and hospital staff with his groaning and yelling. Mindell describes his interaction with the man as follows:

When I saw him, the man was lying in his hospital bed moaning and shouting out something that no one could understand. I groaned with him, "ohhh, oooh, wow, yeah." After about 20 minutes, his muffled shouts became distinguishable words. John, who had not said a word to anyone in days, or uttered a complete sentence in 6 months, now said "yeah…wow…no…yeah…oh".

After elaborating on and extending the sounds and words that John was making, Arny began to distinguish more words. John was talking about a big ship coming for him, and then yelled that he was not getting on that ship. "No man – not me! I'm not getting on that ship. That ship's … going on … vacation. I gotta get up at eight in the morning and go to work!" The conversation goes on:

Arny invites the man to take a good look and say who is driving the ship. John replies that it is angels who are driving. Arny asks John to check out how much it costs

---

[4] Mindell, Arnold (2008, p.14). *Coma: The Dreambody Near Death*

to get on the ship and John replies with amazement that it costs nothing. "It's a free trip" says Arny. "Have you ever had a vacation?" When John responds in the negative, Arny says, "Listen man, you never had a vacation. You're a working man. You should consider a little trip. If you don't like it, you can come back. If you like it, then you can just keep going". John replies, "Yeah ... yeah. Vacation, to the Bahamas, Ba ... ha ... mas... hmmm ... no work." With that John quietened down, closed his eyes and went to sleep. When Arny returned to check on him a half hour later, the nurse reported that John had just died. The old man had decided to go on vacation.

One central question confronting us, during both living and dying, is how we relate to disturbance. Disturbance is so often seen as something that should be eradicated, kept out, or subdued. Of course, disturbance is often uncomfortable and unfamiliar, bringing many of us to a place of irritation or fear, conjuring up experiences of helplessness and disempowerment. The more unknown the experience, the more nervous we may become, attempting to ignore it or run away from it. Disturbance is something we try our hardest to avoid. It is disruptive, challenging, uncomfortable, and often demands change. Body symptoms, dreams, relationship issues, environmental events, and so on, will stalk us until we can embrace them as harbingers of something new and useful to us.

Most of us tend to resist change and do not do so well in adapting to something new. However, if we can embrace disturbance with a recognition that it brings something meaningful for us, that actually the problem itself may have the solution within it, we may be able to find the richness it offers for our lives and deaths. Death is the ultimate disturbance for many in that it strips us of our personal identity and brings huge change, something that we as humans usually resist and fear.

Writing about this, I am reminded of the ancient practise of alchemy, in which base material is looked at as an opportunity to discover gold. Alchemy is thought to be the forerunner of modern chemistry, holding the belief that gold can be made from base metals through a cooking process. Before the 16th century, physics and psychology were all part of same science (Alchemy). While the metals did not actually produce gold, the alchemist him/herself went through a process of transformation, closely aligned to an internal developmental process through which greater self-knowledge emerged. This was seen to be the gold. Instead of fixed solid states, emphasis was on process, the recognition that indeed everything changes and flows.

Personal Identity and Death

At various stages of life, we identify ourselves in a certain way based on what is known and familiar to us. Parts of ourselves are closer to this identity, while other parts are less known or outside of awareness. Our everyday identity is often shaken up and transformed by situations and experiences that happen to us, often in a surprising or unexpected way. Some of these are more acute, visiting us suddenly and then leaving quickly (acute illnesses, accidents, relationship break-ups, environmental upheavals). Others last for longer periods of time, or recur in patterns contributing to the unfolding of a greater understanding of why we exist and what our inherent natures are (chronic symptoms, childhood and recurring dreams, repeating patterns in the choices we make in our work and relationship lives). The involuntary process of aging keeps changing our sense of self and the way we can show up in the world. Terminal illness and the various stages of the dying process are perhaps the most threatening to our personal identity, and it is during these phases of life, that we are most challenged in facing all that this process brings.

As personal identity transforms, and what has been known falls away, we can observe that the person going through terminal phases takes on a different reality. A process of dis-identification occurs. Words spoken, gestures made, physical appearance, all become unfamiliar and hard to relate to. It seems that the person is in a "different world", often hard to track and understand. Some consider that as death approaches we enter another form of ourselves, a far-out state of consciousness that has a different frame of reference to the one we are accustomed to. In Greek mythology, as we near death, we stand at the crossroads waiting for something to guide us in a direction. We are no longer who we have been, nor are we yet who we are to become, but exist in a limbic realm with an as yet unrecognized reality[5]. Something else begins to replace who we have been during life.

---

[5] von Franz (1986) *On Dreams and Death*

Although many of the experiences near death can be challenging and/or disturbing, they can also be uplifting (as described in the example of *The Big Ship*). During this great time of transformation, if we can recognize or identify with what is emerging, death can be a fulfilling passage. Those who attend the dying can be of great help in noticing and making useful the various experiences that visit the dying, helping them in turn to gain awareness of the path opening up for them. How to be a support here and ways to do this are mentioned later in following chapters.

We might well ask, "Why the interest in working further with those in deeply altered experiences during illness and nearing death?"

We know a lot more now about dying. There have been many stories published of near death experiences from people who have come out of comatose states. They have reported what it was like for them and the many unusual occurrences they met in other "worlds"[6]. In some cases, patients were also aware of events happening in the room in which they were lying. The latest scientific research also validates that although patients in coma or in the dying process appear to be without communication and unable to receive communication, recordings of actual brain activity show that there is response to others. Believing in the rich inner life of the patient and acknowledging that to them is a great support for their own experience.

---

[6] Parnia, S; Gutkind, L; Alexander, E.

Different ways of approaching the dying through joining with them, reflecting and framing what the observer notices, and interacting with them physically are found to bring relief and insight for those in the dying process. We can provide assistance so that the person can go further and complete processes in whatever way is needed. Added awareness can be illuminating, even fun. Death can be a wonderful learning time for everyone.

How do we support the Patient's process?

• By helping the patient to get in touch with what is happening on the inside and increasing their awareness of this

• Believing in the patient's experience and its meaning (the teleological perspective which finds usefulness in what presents)

• Supporting them to go further with what is happening for them

• Assisting them to make life and death decisions

• Using the concept of *deep democracy*[7], through which all experience, pleasant or disturbing, is supported in a way that honours and respects it.

This can happen in a number of ways.

Physically - Helping them to become aware of their breath and internal rhythm- amplifying their physical signals no matter how minimal.

Emotionally - picking up on the feeling atmosphere present for them and supporting and encouraging it.

---

[7] Mindell, A. (1992). *The Leader as Martial Artist*

Dreaming - Using fantasy and imagination to help them dream further and follow their visions.

Communication – Creating a binary communication system using signals that are already present.

Attention and Awareness

In everyday lives and situations we are usually unaware of attending to the array of signals and information that impinges on us. We learn to pay attention and take in information that aids us in such basic things as survival on one level, and on others, information that benefits us in relationships, navigating in our work and family lives, and generally assisting us in creating a place for ourselves in the world. We are bombarded in an ongoing way by visual and auditory cues, many of which we relegate to the margins of our awareness. We usually maintain one point of reference from which we view and engage in our world and life. A shift in this point often brings a new way of attending that allows us to enter other layers of perception, or out-of-ordinary states of experience. It is when we attend to usually marginalized signals that we can pick up additional information about both our and others' experience.

Signals and Channels

Signals are pieces of information that we perceive or experience. There are signals that are more obvious, more familiar or known to us. There are other signals that are further from our awareness, or more subtle and unknown. Caregivers, nurses, and helpers may approach signals from different perspectives according to what they've been taught to look for. From a medical model viewpoint, we might interpret a signal such as a fever as a sign of danger needing immediate attention. From another perspective though, a fever may bring information about heating up, being fiery in relationship, more intense, etc. We may look at the fever as a symbolic representation of an underlying phenomenon that needs attending to. The meaning we get from signals differs according to the unique process of the individual, our approach, and the context the patient is in. Part of the work we practice with the dying or comatose, is picking up on signals we notice and helping the patient to become aware of them. We bring attention to them without interpretation, amplify them, and unfold them until some meaning or usefulness is found within them. We are following a teleological perspective, in which all information is viewed as being useful or meaningful in some way. We trust that as we unfold a signal some information or essential experience will emerge from it that can facilitate or enlighten the journey of the dying.

We also attend to these because they allow us to join with the patient and help them with their awareness of what they are experiencing. This both enables the ill, comatose or dying individual to feel met, and also helps them to follow their own experience. In some cases, following a signal can also bring a process to completion when new insight is gained and a life/death lesson learned.

The kinds of signals that are focused on include movements, posture, skin colour, temperature, sounds, breath, changes in pupil size, facial expression, direction of gaze and many more. Sometimes patients close to death or in vegetative states surprise us with sudden flickers of movement in different parts of the body, or unexpected sounds or grimaces. All of these signals are gateways into a deeper layer of experience. If we notice them, bring attention to them and then support them to unfold further, they often bring numinous and deeply felt experience. In the second part of this manual, you will find guiding exercises to help you pick up and unravel signals in yourself and in those you accompany.

Let's read on now to the next chapter in which we talk more about supporting and going further with clients' experiences through the use of attention, signal awareness and amplification.

Chapter 2

The Structure and Flow of Process

*I would love to live life like the river flows
carried by the surprise of its own unfolding.*
- John O' Donohue

Following on from our explanation of the use of attention and signal awareness, in this chapter we will focus on the structure of process, as well as the skills and techniques that guide us in unfolding and completing a process.

As mentioned in Chapter 1, death is a major disturber. One reason why we might struggle with death is that generally in Western culture we keep it separate from life and avoid thinking of it. Death challenges our personal identity and may confront us with parts of ourselves not yet lived or still unknown. The dying process itself can have many unknown or disturbing elements that can be terrifying for those dying and their caregivers. These may include confusion, hallucinations or visions, anxiety and moods. In this next section you will learn skills and techniques to navigate these experiences and make them useful for the person who is dying. In considering these aspects of oneself that are not well known, or that are disturbing to us, we are expanding our identities to encompass previously marginalized information and experience.

One of the basic structures we find in a process focuses on the way in which we normally identify ourselves in everyday life, i.e. our primary identify. There are things in life that we can say are "me". There are also things that are further away from how I experience myself, are more unknown, even disturbing, and are viewed as "not me". For example, today I identify myself as a New Zealander, an older woman, a stepmother and step-grandmother, a sister and half-sister to my siblings, an aunt, friend, psychotherapist, a teacher and right now, a writer. I consider myself to be well educated, generally healthy and liking to eat well and keep fit.

Then last night I had a dream. In the dream I had parked my car in the middle of the road. As the dream unfolded, I was taken to a group in a building where a crazy dentist started telling us off. From the perspective of believing that all parts of the dream are a reflection of the dreamer, the crazy dentist, as an aspect of myself, is someone I don't identify with and know little about. He is the more disturbing and unknown part of the dream. Also I don't normally park my car in the middle of the road!

As well as in dreams, things we consider to be "not me" or disturb us in some way, also appear in body symptoms, chronic illness, fantasies, altered states of consciousness, relationship conflicts and world events. In everyday life we normally try to avoid these experiences, ignore them, dislike them, fight them or push them away. However, from the teleological and deeply democratic perspective, these disturbances are viewed as potentially meaningful and important to us in our growth and development, bringing information that can enhance our sense of who we are, our wellbeing and happiness.

Take a few moments to consider the following:

• *How do you identify yourself these days? Gender, age, race, education, wealth, health, work, relationships, other.*

• *What things would you consider to be not you? In other words, what things or experiences disturb you or happen to you? These could be dreams or dream–like experiences, body symptoms, other people, relationship conflicts, accidents.*

• *Choose one of these and notice what kind of energy or quality is held in that. How could that be useful to you?*

• *Make a few notes.*

Next you will find some concepts and theoretical ideas to consider when unfolding process, either in yourself or in others whom you may be supporting.

Metaskills

Metaskills[8] are the feeling attitudes and belief systems that accompany us when we are in interaction with ourselves and with others. In other words, do we tend to be mostly compassionate and understanding, or are we more evaluative or critical. Do we have an existential or spiritual belief that influences our relationship style and conviction about what needs to happen? These background attitudes become apparent when we are attempting to intervene with another, or to relate to someone who is outside of our usual framework. It is helpful to identify the metaskills that are generally with us, and how they may lead us in our interactions, especially when we are in the role of supporter, caretaker or helper. Once we know these, we might want to develop some further and curtail others, or even introduce metaskills that we don't already have.

One of the reasons we may find it difficult to accompany and assist someone at end of life and beyond, is the fear of doing something wrong or of being insensitive at an emotional time. At these times, let us not forget that we do have innate qualities and attitudes that we bring with us that are helpful. Feeling attitudes such as compassion, empathy, curiosity, courage, patience, playfulness, openness to what is happening without preconceived ideas, and a welcoming attitude, are important and encouraged. Sometimes our own belief system or spiritual practice will further enhance the development of these qualities and attitudes and enable us to be present with our own dying and that of others.

---

[8] Mindell, Amy (1995) *Metaskills: The Spiritual Art of Therapy*

Being aware of what metaskills we hold within us and bring to others, will enable us to use these more consciously in order to meet patients or loved ones in a way that supports their views and beliefs. We will also be able to identify the areas in which we might need to grow in order not to get polarized against the belief systems that others hold for themselves. This becomes particularly important when grappling with patients and family members who hold different, or opposite, views to the ones we value.

Doorways into Experience

Following a process rests on our ability to find and pick up signals. Signals are bits of information. They include things such as a grin, a sigh, a frown, a grimace, body movements, eye movements, crying, laughing, a tone of voice or a sound. Signals are doorways into experiences. Some signals are obvious while others are subtler or minimal. As caregivers, nurses, or helpers we may approach signals from different perspectives according to what we have been trained to look for. From a medical perspective we might interpret a signal, a grimace for example, as a sign of the patient being in pain. Those in attendance will therefore consider some kind of medication to reduce that. From a process-oriented perspective however, this signal may indicate something completely different, either an expression of, or a reaction to, an internal experience; or to something that the patient is aware of in his immediate environment. If we go further in drawing attention to this signal, and then amplify it increasing the grimace and facial expression, a completely different figure or experience may pop out of it, for example a figure or face of a wizened, ancient being who may hold a completely different view of dying to that of the patient. This view could in turn bring more wisdom and a deeper insight for the patient him/herself.

Supporting those who are dying involves noticing signals and helping the person become aware of them through amplifying them (see below), dreaming into them (see Chapter 4) and helping the person find meaning in them. In doing that, we are hoping we can unfold some less known information or essential experience for them. The meaning found when signals are unravelled differs for each individual. Signals express uniquely for each of us. We try to avoid interpreting them, but rather enter the experience they bring in order to find meaning or insight.

I was sitting with a patient whom I will call Pam. She was experiencing something no one could understand or relate to. Her carer told me that Pam looked like she was in a trance as her eyes were glazed over, not seeing or talking to anyone. She had been like this for several hours. When I visited her, I noticed how she kept looking up at the corner of the room by the window. She nodded when I told her I was there but her gaze remained on the corner. I gently encouraged her to trust what was happening and to follow what she was seeing. Again she nodded and shorty after a tear ran down her cheek and she began to cry. Her eyes then shifted and she looked at me. She told me she had seen her mother who had died several years ago. Her mother was telling her to be brave and that she would see her soon. Pam found comfort in this vision. From then on she seemed to be more at peace with herself and what was happening to her.

My following Pam's experience (her signal of looking up), and supporting her to both notice it and go further into it, tweaked her own awareness of it. She was then able to recognize and explore it further. This brought her an encouraging and helpful message from her dead mother.

Going through the Doorway

When you have noticed a signal it is important to identify where it is located and how it is making itself known. Is the person experiencing an emotion or inner body feeling, expressing a thought, hearing something or making a sound, seeing an image, making a movement, experiencing a relationship conflict, or is there something happening in the wider environment? The person will give us clues as to how they perceive or express what is happening to them. These are doorways, *dream doors* into deeper experience. For example, in the story above, Pam was looking up at the corner of the room when seeing her mother. Looking up gave me the clue that she was seeing an image. I was able to encourage her to go further with that experience which then changed to feelings of sadness and then relief. If her eyes were looking down I would have expected her to be having a body feeling, and if her eyes were looking straight ahead or to the side I would think that she was listening, perhaps hearing a sound or voice[9]. These clues provide us with a way to go into and through the doorway in order to discover what is trying to happen.

So you can see how signals, and how they appear, assist us to establish communication with the dying person even when they are less responsive. Those who are becoming less responsive or are in vegetative states or coma still show signals, but these are subtler and thus often more difficult to notice. In these cases, we need to sharpen our awareness in order to notice the doorways and enter them. By picking up on the signals we notice, and supporting them to go further, we are able to join with the patient in their world of experience and bring that to awareness for them. We also then are able to hold an awareness of the whole process that is trying to happen. Rather than trying to change the person's experience, we acknowledge what is happening for them. Learning how to enter and follow the person's experience using signals and the sensory pathways discussed above, gives us the way forward. We try to avoid interpreting or judging, but rather enter the experience with an open mind. You can also learn more about skills for working with signals and channel experiences in *Coma: A Healing Journey: A guide for families, friends and Helpers.* [10]

---

[9] Bandler & Grinder (1979) *Frogs into Princes: Neuro-linguistic Programming*

[10] Mindell, Amy (1999) *Coma: A Healing Journey: A guide for families, friends and Helpers*

Channels and Sensory-grounded Information

Patients' experiences and perceptions manifest through different sensory modalities. We can observe how information is being expressed in a particular sensory channel through certain signals. Becoming aware of signals in various sensory-oriented channels means we can make interventions that match that channel of expression, facilitating connection with the patient. Different ways of perceiving and expressing are known as channels or sensory pathways. Once recognized, they show us which direction to take in order to go further into the process. In order to go further, it is useful to access *sensory-grounded information*. This means that we obtain information regarding an experience in terms of the way it is sensed or perceived. For example, when we experience pain it is helpful to notice the characteristics of that pain – is it sharp, dull, piercing, throbbing, etc. Obtaining this information brings more awareness to the experience and unfolds the process further by amplifying the nature of that particular experience. Let's say that the patient describes that pain as piercing and as we go further into that, a movement emerges to describe it. Going into the movement and amplifying that, noticing its direction and quality, may bring in a sense of being laser-like and focused. This quality may be really useful to the patient both in the way they attend to and carry out tasks or activities, or in the way they might relate to others.

Exploring signals in the various channels in which they appear is helpful in deepening a process and accessing its meaning. We attend to these because they allow us to join with the patient and help them become conscious of what may lie beneath their awareness that wants to be lived more fully.

We like to divide ways of perceiving and experiencing into the following channels.

Visual

Signals in this channel will appear when looking or seeing is involved. You may notice the eyes looking up or when closed, you may notice the eyeball moving upward under the closed lid. Eyes may also follow somebody in the room or be looking out of the window or at one spot. Verbal content includes "seeing" words. Ways of exploring experiences in the visual channel include colour, shape, size and images. Encouraging the patient to take a "look" will help to amplify the experience in this channel, as well as inviting descriptions of size, colour, shape etc.

Auditory

Signals appear in this channel through sound, voice, verbal content, thoughts, listening to or hearing something, and silence. You may notice that "hearing" or "thinking" words are used. Eyes may look straight ahead or to the side. The head may be leaning to one side with ear cocked as if trying to hear something. Ways of exploring experience in the auditory channel are to encourage the patient to really "listen", to make sounds louder, to hum or sing, or to give words to experience.

Proprioception

Another way of exploring body experiences is through the proprioceptive channel. This means tapping into inner body experiences, feelings, and emotions.

Some somatic experiences may be pain, pressure, temperature. Emotions may include sadness, joy, excitement, fear, etc. How do we recognise proprioceptive signals? We may notice signals such as looking down, hunched body posture, closed eyes, pauses and verbal content that uses "feeling" words. The use of blank access (see chapter 3, p. 26) can be useful in helping the patient to amplify the experience and thus bring more awareness to it. Encouragement to feel that more or to make the feeling bigger, are also ways of amplifying proprioceptive experiences.

Movement

Signals in the movement channel may be obvious or subtle. The movement channel includes all kinds of movement, even those movements we cannot see like throbbing or pulsing, or stillness itself. Other movement signals include:

- Swallowing- most often indicates a thought and is typically related to feeling
- Eyebrows twitching – may indicate an internal visual experience, or effort
- Large or minimal hand/feet /leg movements, turning of the head, muscle contractions in lower jaw, movement of the lips, dilation of the pupils, etc.

Movement can be amplified by encouraging the patient to move even more, to imagine what that movement would become if it could be expressed fully, or to assist in the movement through touch or physical support of the movement.

Relationship

Relationship experiences occur through interaction with others, or even internally in relating to parts of oneself. Relationship signals can be noticed through postures and gestures, e.g. the other's body is turned towards or away from you, the other's gaze is fixed on you, the patient's hand moves towards your own, verbal content may contain reference to others or to relationship issues and/or conflict. Encouraging relationship signals includes saying something about what you notice, supporting the patient to follow the signal further, or if the patient is able, to talk about the relationship.

Now try the following exercise, taking your time with each step.

• Stand up and for a moment focus on your body.

• Notice any movement happening there. This could be a minimal movement such as a twitch or slight movement, or it could be a bigger/more obvious movement.

• Focus on this movement and amplify it (express/move it more/make it bigger) and then make a sound that goes with it.

• Now add an image that goes along with the movement and sound.

• Is there a feeling sense that goes along with this experience?

- Now bring it all together and act it out. Notice if a figure, personality, quality or way of being emerges from this experience.

You have just unfolded a signal using different sensory pathways that you may normally not have been aware of. Make a note of what you found there. How could that be useful to you in your everyday life?

Amplification

So why go further into disturbance when it can be easier to stop what is happening and bring comfort? Of course such things as medication and distracting the attention by following something other than the disturbance are really helpful and necessary at times, especially when someone is in pain. We know though that if an experience is repressed or marginalised it tends to return even more strongly. As mentioned earlier we are also interested in the meaning of what is happening. This is where amplification becomes useful.

In amplifying an experience (just as we did through the exercise above), rather than trying to stop the experience, we support the person to bring more attention to what is happening. Amplification entails bringing more awareness to an experience, getting to know more about it by enlarging or intensifying it, extending it to the whole body, or into other sensory channels of perception, and then integrating it into everyday awareness. As we amplify, the experience seems to take on a life of its own, taking us with it as we follow what emerges. Amplification often includes a shift to different sensory channels, enlarging and rounding out the experience in order to unfold the process further. Amplification brings a non-linear way of burrowing further into the lesser-known aspects that are waiting to be discovered and recognized, bringing an expanded view of the self. When insight into what is trying to emerge is reached, we find that the disturbance is relieved and the patient reaches a new state of experience.

Feedback

We are also able to pick up feedback from the patient to alert us as to whether we are on the right track or not. In the example mentioned earlier where the woman looks up into the corner, Pam gave positive feedback to interventions made, following suggestions and responding with interest. A response that holds energy, even if it is resisting an intervention, may be taken as positive feedback. In other words, there is a "spark" or energetic response indicating that there is more to unfold, even if it seems to go against our attempt to intervene. In some cases we might encounter actual negative feedback, e.g. a patient turning away from us when we enter the room or make a suggestion, or a complete lack of interest in our interventions. There is a "flatness" or lack of response that indicates there is no energy in that direction. It is up to us to notice what kind of responses we get from those we are attempting to join. Even a lack of response, or a minimal reaction, is feedback of some kind. In order to understand more of the patient's process, it can then be up to our own ability to dream into the patient's experience, or to use symbolic thinking in these cases. Please see chapter 4 for more information on *dreaming*.

Pacing the Breath

(See exercise on pacing the breath in Part II)

Pacing the breath is a way of connecting and joining with those who are in the dying process. This technique is especially useful with those who are in a less responsive state or comatose state near death, but generally most people love it and feel very nourished by it. You can even practice this with family members, children, and peers. It is a simple technique, first introduced by Arny and Amy Mindell[11] that includes touch in the least invasive way through placing your hand/s on the wrist, or soles of the feet. In this technique, we are joining with and pacing the natural rhythm of the patient's breath by squeezing the wrist, or pushing against the soles, at each in-breath, and releasing at each out-breath. This can also be used with patients who have a tracheotomy and are on a respirator.

The technique brings the patient's awareness to his or her own breathing pattern and creates the basis for connecting inwardly, harnessing awareness of inner experiences.

Rather than leaving the dying alone in their experience, pacing the breath is a way we can relate to them so that they feel our presence and know we are supporting them in their deep inner experience. This is an effortless experience for the patient through which attention is given by the caregiver without the patient having to respond or relate.

Edges

---

[11] Mindell, Amy (1999) *Coma- A Healing Journey*

At times we may find it difficult to go further through a *dream door* due to a number of reasons. One may be our own patterning in reaction to past trauma or personal history. A second is often fear. Fear to go into something unknown which is unfamiliar and not yet experienced. Another may be the cultural and familial beliefs that we've grown up with, which inhibit and often stop us from going further. These beliefs may have a number of "voices" and manifest as either criticism of ourselves, messages of cultural appropriateness, or as warnings of threat. When any or all of these occur, we find ourselves at an *edge*. An edge is the place between what we identify with as being "me" and what is unknown or less familiar. It is here that we encounter the many belief systems and fears, described above, that stop us from going into the unknown. We may hear ourselves saying, "I can't do this. It is not me" or a critical voice that says, "you are not good enough and will certainly fail here" or even another that says, "nobody will like you if you do that." When this happens it is helpful to take a moment to check in with ourselves and address what is happening internally. In other words, do we want to go along with this critical voice or perhaps say no to it. If the latter we may need to interact with the critical figure or whatever it is that is stopping us from going further, finding out more about it and where it has a hold over us. If we are unable to clear this, talking to someone can help.

Edges are places where we meet parts of ourselves that are marginalised and not yet fully lived. During the dying process, and especially at death, we are likely to meet some big edges face-to-face. Those near death and actively dying, might come up against some big edges and not know how to move forward. Often they need assistance to negotiate an edge. Our understanding of where they may be at in themselves, what edges may have come up for them, and our ability to join with them and guide them according to signals that emerge, may encourage them to cross these edges and engage in the lesser-known aspects appearing to them. This process of encountering less-known parts of the self, can be immensely relieving to the dying person, and may bring deeper insight that sheds light on the path they are taking, freeing the person from anxiety, fear or uncertainty.

As death draws nearer, however, and the person enters a more altered-like state where they connect to sentient or spiritual realms, they enter a place that goes beyond having to navigate edges. At this juncture, they often lose touch with everyday awareness. We can assist them by being present with them, supporting and encouraging them to go further with what is happening. As you read on to the next chapter, we will be introducing you to methods that can be of assistance to those in far-out or altered states of consciousness where edges are not apparent, and another kind of approach is needed.

Chapter 3

Far-Out and Altered States of Consciousness

Logic will get you from A to B. Imagination will take you everywhere.

\- Albert Einstein

As most patients go further into the dying experience or get closer to death, their usual way of perceiving and experiencing goes through a change. Consensus reality and everyday identity as they have known it are no longer so prevalent in their awareness and it seems they operate from a different perspective. On the way to death we often go through various coma-like and near-death states and experiences, which manifest through the body and also put us into dreamy and altered levels of consciousness. It is within these that we can access teachings for both life and death.

There are many reports from people who have gone through near-death and comatose experiences[12] where they describe the transformed way in which they experience their inner and outer environments, their perception of others, and the way in which their awareness functions. Their perceptions of the material world become hazier and clouded, holding an ethereal, subtle or other-worldly aspect. As the patient meets material substance, imaginal figures, dream-like objects, and essential tendencies and energies, they come into contact with aspects of themselves or their environments previously unknown, perhaps only met in dreams. Often our loved ones or patients, in these deeper processes, are unable to verbalize or describe what they are experiencing. We may be able to catch brief sentences, disjointed words, exclamations or other sounds, or even more subtle signals like slight movements or a blink, but it becomes difficult from the outside to understand or make contact with them. In this chapter, we will be describing the ways in which these states of consciousness manifest, how they might be supported and how we may be able to make contact with those in more deeply altered experiences.

With near-death and vegetative-like states, the usual inference is that there is no awareness in the patient, although this is now disputed by recent research. On our side we believe there is awareness that we can in part connect with. As we usually marginalize these unusual experiences in ourselves in everyday existence, we find it hard to conceive that states like this even exist. The more we can get in touch with these experiences in

---

[12] Alexander, S; Gutkind, L; Parnia, E.

ourselves, the more we can support the patient in theirs. It therefore becomes important for those around the patient (if they want to get a sense of where the patient is in their inner world) to explore what it may be like to be in a far-out state, something that may previously have gone unnoticed. Developing self-awareness, being in touch with our own feelings, our own beliefs, values, and ethics and what experiences lie outside of our usual states of consciousness becomes important in being able to join with the patient, as we are then able to guide the patient by understanding their inner experience from our own. We say more about how to do this further on in this chapter.

Rather than leave the person alone to fend for themselves, we can provide assistance so that the person can go further and complete processes in whatever way is needed. This includes, finishing off stuff like incomplete relationships with family members and loved ones; concrete tasks they are concerned about; assisting them to go further in their process to bring more of a sense of fulfilment or completion; supporting them to live their last days more fully like perhaps they have never done before; or assisting them to die. We can help them to get in touch with what is happening on the inside and bring their awareness to it, supporting them to go further with what is trying to gain recognition and become known.

As the patient enters and proceeds along the terminal stages of life, we notice that there is a continuum of various states of consciousness. This ranges from a consensus reality identity (their everyday identity as it has been) through various stages of altered awareness as the person moves away from the person they have known to be "themselves". It is here that the patient begins to tap into more unknown and "far-out" states, ultimately experiencing comatose-like, near-death and dying states of awareness. As the person moves along this progression, we may begin to understand less of what they are encountering, both in their inner and outer perception. However, as mentioned before, we do have some access to these states through the various signals and sensory channel experiences that manifest. It is through these that we can begin to enter and join their worlds. We have talked about signals in chapter 2 – how to notice and amplify them, thus bringing more attention to them – and you will find further pointers and exercises in addition to those already mentioned, in the second part of this book, to help you in finding ways to join and support the dying person.

As we go further in this chapter, we discuss a variety of tools that can be used in meeting the dying on the level of their experience, or in the state of consciousness that exists for them. If we are able to do this, we are then able to hold an awareness both for the patient and ourselves, of the larger process which is playing out. We are generally engaging on at least three different dimensions with the dying person. As mentioned, these weave in and out of each other as the patient enters different states of consciousness, almost as though visiting parallel worlds, each with its own ways of perceiving and experiencing. We give a short breakdown of these below and ways in which you might identify them. Each defines a way of relating and engaging.

Consensus Reality

The way in which we normally identify ourselves. A patient may identify herself as a wife and mother. She may be an artist. She also now identifies as having cancer. We can agree on this – there is concrete evidence. We can also connect with her in terms of this identity in that we can talk with her in a familiar, concrete way about her art, her children, and the fact that she has contracted cancer.

Dreamland

We find a lot of information here that is useful for the ongoing process in addition to waking us up to parts of ourselves we're not usually aware of. Here we find experiences underlying consensus reality that express themselves through signals, metaphor, dreams, fantasy and delusions. These are usually outside of our known identity and in addition we may find them disturbing or mysterious. The images, body experiences and atmospheres that we meet here are usually on the fringes of our awareness. These experiences may also be outside of the temporal and spatial frameworks that we know in consensus reality. Our patient from above may have a fantasy that she is in another time and place. She might be engaged there in an action or task that is not present in her everyday world at that moment. Such experiences are not so easy to talk about, and are often marginalized as being "not real", in that the patient is "confused" or "hallucinating".

Essence

Here we encounter subtle pre-verbal tendencies that manifest through essence-like experiences (usually subtle body feelings and movements) that are very hard to put into words. As the patient gets further along in the dying process, these kinds of experiences are entered more frequently and it becomes more difficult to connect in the verbal channel. Here we begin to rely more on very subtle signals like minimal sounds and movements, and the use of dreaming and blank access interventions discussed below.

Here is a case example that illustrates the process when working with the three levels described above.

Jill, an 80 year-old, was determined to stay in her own home for as long as possible during her aging process. Unfortunately, she became too ill and fragile to look after herself and had to move into a Residential Care facility (Consensus Reality). *Leaving her home was traumatic for her. For several weeks she complained about the care she received and longed to go home. When I visited her she looked distressed. She was in pain and struggling* (Consensus Reality) *to come to terms with her impending death. Her family was concerned and felt bad that they could not comply with her wishes.*

Jill also told me that she wanted to go home. I asked her to tell me about home (Dreamland) *and what that meant for her. Her eyes looked up as she began to describe her garden* (Dreamland). *She said it had a cherry tree in the middle of the lawn and the most beautiful daisies and pansies of all colours around the edge of the lawn. She talked about her kowhai tree and how the Tui birds loved it* (Dreamland). *As she spoke I noticed her face became slightly pink and her voice started to soften and become a little dreamy. I encouraged her to go further and imagine being in the garden now and take a good look at all she can see and hear there. She smiled and went further into her experience. She was vey quiet so I supported her to take all the time she needed to be there. After a few moments I encouraged her to go further and feel the essential quality of the garden, the essence of her experience, the deep feeling sense of home* (Essence). *I supported Jill by encouraging her to make a small movement with her hand, or let a sound arise, that went along with how she was feeling. She made a slow minimal movement with her right hand and began to softly hum. I asked her if there was a word to describe this experience. She thought for a moment then said: "Peace"* (Essence).

We talked about what she had experienced in her garden and that whenever she felt the need she could go "home" in her imagination.

Below we suggest some techniques for you as helpers or family members of the patient in order to provide you with some useful tools in being with your patient or loved one based on an understanding of the above levels.

Believing in the Presenting State

Believing in the state that presents itself is very important. This means we need to be sufficiently fluid to leave our consensus reality world behind and join with the patient in their experience, trying to dream about and access the deeper states that they are experiencing. Once we understand more about what is trying to happen there we can support its meaning for the patient and attempt to make a link between the patient's usual/past primary identity and this less familiar state. As mentioned above, we can pick up on the patient's experience by noticing body signals, attending to verbal and auditory cues, and using our own capacity to dream along with the patient (see p.27). Here are some additional suggestions as to what to look for:

- Respiratory rate - Notice whether it is erratic or regular, labored or light, deep or shallow.
- Eye movements, dilations, eyelid twitches, flickers
- Skin changes – flushing, temperature, goosebumps (cutis anserina)
- Body language - posture, movements of limbs, twitches in fingers or toes, muscle tension.
- Vocalizations, coughs, sneezes, unidentifiable noises, unintelligible speech
- Atmospheres, moods, your own reactions and feelings, images that come to you.

This work takes time when you start doing it as you need time to feel yourself into the other's state, to pace the person's breathing, and to notice the signals and movements. After a while it becomes a second language, more natural to you, and can be used in any small or large interactions.

Supporting the Patient to Believe in their Experience
Even though the patient might not be apparently listening to you and others, or communicating much at all, and may seem to be completely out of touch with the kinds of experiences we usually identify with, it is still

possible to help them become aware of what is happening for them and to validate those experiences. The first step in this is joining with them as we have described above. The next piece is to assist them to become aware of aspects of what might be going on for them internally, and then to support their trust of, and belief in their individual process. Like many of us, those near death or in a coma, will tend to marginalize experiences that are uncomfortable or unknown, might even be afraid of them, but if we can help them to believe in these, it is possible then to find the deeper meaning and direction for their path.

We are basically assisting the patient to:

• Get in touch with what is happening on the inside thus increasing their awareness of their inner world

• Unfold their experiences by amplification of signals

• Believe in their experience and its meaning

• Go further with what is happening for them and make it useful

• Make life and death decisions

Important tools and skills for the helper/family member are the following:

Metaskills[13] (previously discussed in chapter 2)

These are the feeling attitudes and belief systems that are an inherent part of us and that we bring in when in interaction. For example, our attitudes around death and

---

[13] Mindell, Amy (1995) *Metaskills: The Spiritual Art of Therapy*

dying; our spiritual beliefs; where we place emphasis in our interactions – patience or pressure to reach a goal; do we have compassion and empathy in being with the dying person; are we playful or more serious ... and so on.

Metacommunication

The ability to make "meta" comments on what we perceive is happening in any given moment. For example, when noticing a deep breath in the other we may say, "that looked like a deep breath"; or when someone turns away from you to say, "I see you turn away"; or on feeling sadness to say, "I feel sad right now" and so on. Metacommunication is a very versatile and valuable tool and can be applied in many moments in a process to keep awareness of what is happening for all involved. We may view our role here as that of awareness keeper.

Metaphor

We use symbols and metaphor in order to go deeper with the patient in their process. (See Chapter 4).

Blank Access

Blank access provides us with a way of intervening with the client that is non-invasive, non-directive and avoids making assumptions about the patient's experience. Using blank access helps us to avoid interpretations and labelling. Signs and signals may easily be misinterpreted. Blank access leaves an opening for the patient to have their experience without us naming it for them. We merely draw awareness to something without defining, interpreting, or making boundaries for it. The patient, in an altered state of consciousness, has his or her own inner experience which we often can't perceive directly. Blank access therefore supports the patient to follow what is happening for them without our naming it specifically. It leaves things open for the patient to pick up in a way that best serves them.

Examples of blank access interventions:
- "Notice what is happening and follow that"
- "Yes … I hear that sound / see that movement"
- "Believe in whatever you notice inside yourself"
- A simple "ah ha" or "hmmm"
- A light touch on a part that may be moving with a comment about noticing the movement

Dreaming

Joining with the other through dreaming about what is happening for them and using one's own dreaming experience as a barometer. Knowing something of their personal history, their likes and tendencies, can be helpful here. Becoming aware of what comes up for you personally in being with them and seeing that as part of the field phenomenon around them, being reflected in all aspects of the field, including oneself. (See more about field phenomena in Chapter 7). Your own dreaming in terms of images, body sensations, and feeling reactions that come up for you, may also be helpful in understanding where the patient or loved one may be at.

An important part of being able to work with mythical processes and dreams is our capacity to enter dreaming. Remember when we were kids and we were able to create fantasies, dreaming about all sorts of things while we were awake. Objects and people could take on remarkable shapes, forms, voices and act in wonderful ways. Here again, we want to cultivate this capacity in ourselves so that we can enter the dream/ing to join all of those figures, characters and energies both in ourselves and in others. I often think of the development of this capacity as the growth of a muscle that needs to be maintained and nourished.

The *Assemblage Point* is the point of reference from which we usually view and engage in our world and life[14]. A shift in this point often brings a new way of attending that allows us to perceive events, figures or objects in a non-ordinary way. Here are some ways we can access *dreaming:*

• Allowing awareness to become clouded and dreamy – sensing and perceiving from that state.

• Imagining being the other. Entering into their way of being; seeing through their eyes; having their feelings and entering their inner experiences.

• Entering other levels of experience such as dreamland figures, and essence-like experiences

• Putting our usual selves aside to become somebody else, a dream figure, another quality or energy.

---

[14] Castanedas, C. (1975) *The Eagle's Gift*

- Being open to the path indicated by signals, synchronicities, and tendencies rather than being goal-oriented.

You will find an exercise to cultivate your capacity to *dream* in Part II of this book.

The use of your *Dreaming* muscle will enrich your relationship to yourself, as well as facilitate your interactions with others and especially with those near death.

Binary Communication

We may often find ourselves wanting to ask patients in deep vegetative or comatose states questions, such as: Are you in pain? Shall we turn off your life support? Do you want to come out of your coma? Are you afraid of what may lie ahead? And so on. A process-oriented approach offers an effective way to acquire answers to questions using a communication system that enables the patient to respond "yes" to questions asked if the answer is in the affirmative. If there is a "no" to the question, the patient gives no response. This system is known as a binary communication system.

Setting up binary communication means identifying a repeated signal from the patient, assisting the patient to become aware of the signal, and encouraging them to use it to communicate in response to a question. The first step in this process is to identify a recurring signal that presents itself on an ongoing basis. This could be a twitch of an eyebrow, a blink of an eye, slight movement of a finger, hand, leg, or foot, or any other signal that makes itself known to you through ongoing observation of the patient.

Once the signal is identified we need to help the patient to become aware of it, to notice how the signal manifests, and what it feels like for the patient. We also want to support them to repeat the signal, and we can do this in some of the ways we have already described. If we notice a slight movement of a finger, for example, we can bring attention to that by verbally describing it, touching the finger and assisting it to move, amplifying the movement by helping to make it bigger or more global (moving the whole hand), and bringing the patient's other hand to feel the movement. We can also encourage the patient to use awareness to notice how this is experienced internally, e.g. "notice what it feels like inside you when you move your finger." In order to integrate awareness of the signal, we may want to practice this many times, before the patient is ready to use it as a communication tool. No matter what signal we decide to go with, we can use the same methods described above for raising awareness of it for the patient. Please be aware that the more present and obvious the signal is, the easier it will be to facilitate awareness of it[15].

Lastly, we will want to attempt to use that signal to respond in an affirmative manner to a question asked. Remember that making the movement signifies a "yes" response. There will be no response needed for a "no"

---

[15] Mindell, Amy (1999) *Coma-A Healing Journey: A guide for families, friends and Helpers*

answer. Leaning in close to the patient, and speaking directly to them (into their ear if possible if comatose), begin by asking simple questions like, "are you comfortable" "may I sit next to you" "would you like the window open" and so on. If the signal is being used by the patient to communicate, you may then progress to more specific questions relevant to the patient's treatment, e.g. "are you in pain" "would you like medication for the pain" "would you like a massage" and ultimately, "would you prefer that you be taken off life support". We can also ask questions related to the person's current altered states, for example, "are you having a good time in there"?

If there is no response, say, "I see no response. You may be saying no to that question". Or if you see that part moving, say, "I see your eyelid moving, that must be a yes to my question".

We need to keep in mind that the patient's responses may be delayed due to brain injury, medication effects, effects of illness, and the altered state in which the patient finds themselves. Always try a number of times on consecutive days to make sure the response is an accurate one before you use it as a bona fide communication. If unsure whether the response is accurate, repeat it or go away for a while, come back (even the next day) and try again.

Here is an example of how to use this communication system with a patient.

I was called in by a family for consultation regarding their mother, Anne, aged 80, who had suffered a severe stroke and who was in a deep coma. Anne had been hospitalized for the past 2 weeks and was on life support. The family did not know what Anne's wishes would be in this situation and called me in to help. I spent some time talking with the family as a whole to gauge the general direction that they were considering. They wanted the best for their mother and were in agreement that removing her from life support would be in her best interests. However, they were uncertain if this would be the right direction for her, and whether this would be something that their mother would also want.

I visited Anne on a number of different occasions, worked with her movements and inner process, supporting her to follow what felt right for her. Members of the family were often with me in the hospital room. As I spent time with her I noticed that there was a recurring flicker of her one eyelid. I brought attention to this, lightly touching the eyelid and simulating the flicker for her so she would be more aware of this movement. I also placed her fingers lightly on my eyelid so I could demonstrate the experience for her. I then invited her to repeat the flicker if she was able. She was, although it did take her some time to respond, and then hesitantly. After testing this a number of times I then began to introduce simple questions, inviting her to move her eyelid if the answer to my questions was a "yes". She was able to do this. I explained that if she wanted to respond with a "no", she needn't move at all. (Sometimes there was no response at all and this clearly indicated a "no" response). We now had developed a method of communicating and it was time to consult with the family once again as to their wishes. I wanted to make sure that the whole family was in agreement about the next step we were to take, namely, asking Anne if she wanted to be taken off life support.

The first time I put the question to her the whole family was gathered around letting Anne know that they were in favour of any direction she wanted to take. They told her that they loved her very much and wanted to support her in any way that was right for her. I explained clearly to Anne that we were going to ask her an important question and she could indicate her answer in the affirmative by moving her eyelid in the way we had already established. I asked, "do you want to be taken off life support"? Anne's eyelid fluttered. We waited for about ten minutes before putting the question to her again. There was a clear indication of a "yes" response. Over the next few days we continued to periodically ask this question (as well as others) to make sure that the perceived response was initiated by Anne volitionally. The family communicated their decision to the doctors in charge of the case and all agreed to remove Anne from life support.

The day finally came. Anne was disconnected from all devices keeping her alive. The family gathered around the bedside, holding Anne's hand, telling family stories of experiences together, and singing Anne's favourite songs to her. After some time, Anne died peacefully with a smile on her lips.

Throughout this chapter we have demonstrated a number of ways in which far-out and altered states may be experienced and expressed by the patient, as well as perceived and joined by ourselves. In the second part of this book, you will find exercises that will assist you in getting to know more about your own altered-like experiences, and in practicing the methods and attitudes described in this chapter.

In the next chapter we go further into exploring specific kinds of altered-like experiences such as those found in Delirium and Dementia.

Chapter 4

Whose Reality is this Anyway?

In the words of a Zen poem - At dusk the cock announces dawn, at midnight, the bright sun.

— Fritjof Capra

In addition to the altered kinds of experiences we've mentioned in the last chapter, there are at least two other, more specific forms in which altered-like experiences manifest. These are delirium and dementia.

Most of us have a really hard time making sense of these expressions, let alone being able to join or connect with them. Because we are unable to piece together the verbal content that can also go along with relatively bizarre behaviours associated with these presentations, we tend to pathologize them, view them as "crazy" or incomprehensible, or as making no sense at all. Yet, we are able to work with them in very much the same ways that we have already described. In picking up on signals and channel experiences, mirroring and amplifying these expressions, following metaphors and dream-like manifestations, we are able to join with loved ones or patients and support or guide them in their unique experiences. Even if we cannot find any overt meaning in them, we still believe that they have value, and if processed in the ways described, can enhance underlying directions and ways of being for those who experience them. Let's take a look at how process-oriented techniques can be applied to the following.

Delirium

We may all experience delirium or acute alterations in consciousness at some time in our lives. Delirium can occur during high fevers, as a result of medication or aggressive treatments such as chemotherapy. They can also occur during major change, or through infections, kidney or liver failure, nutritional problems, and may be connected to brain tumours, lack of oxygen, or occur at the end of life. In fact, delirium is known to be one of the most common altered state experiences at end of life. 80%-90% of dying people experience some delirium. Yet we are generally surprised by it and ill prepared in interacting with it. It is something we get nervous about or fear because we mostly don't know what is going on or how to deal with it.

There are certain signs that we can look for that will inform us when someone is experiencing delirium. Symptoms include confusion, delusions, paranoia, hallucinations, incoherent speech, anxiety and restlessness, memory impairment, inability to orient to time and space, and sleep disturbances.

From a biomedical perspective, delirium is assessed in terms of hypoactivity, that is when the person is sleepy and withdrawn, or hyperactivity when the person is agitated, hallucinating or delusional. There can also be a mixture of both.

The usual treatment plan is to use medication to either reverse the state or sedate the person. Sometimes psychotropic drugs are used. These drugs tend to have a restraining and dampening influence and may keep the patient sedated until death. The main focus is to keep the person comfortable and safe. Staff are trained to reassure families, to create a quiet and well-lit atmosphere, to have familiar people around, and a clock on the wall to orient the person to everyday time and space.

Delirium is interpreted in a variety of ways depending on different cultural perspectives. For example, in India delirium is viewed as an opportunity for a life review. In Western countries it is usually pathologized. If it were not that the person was going through the dying process, the patient could well be placed in a mental health unit.

In his seminal book, *Hallucinations*, Oliver Sacks[16] talks about his experience with a man he calls Mr. P who is dying of kidney failure. He is described by staff as "talking nonsense". Sacks is at first also unable to make sense of what Mr. P is saying. "He was talking non-stop with wild associated leaps from one thought to another". However, the more Sacks listened the more he understood. The longer he spent with Mr. P, the more he began to see that Mr. P was re-living events and passions

---

[16]Sachs, Oliver (2012)

from a long and varied life. It was like "being privy to a dream". As Sacks listened, Mr. P became less agitated and clearer, as if having someone to listen to him assisted him to keep going and attempt to bring his story to a conclusion. He died soon after having finished the story.

As with other altered and extreme states, delirium, from a process-oriented perspective, is viewed as a portal (entry) into dreamland, providing a quick way to access new information. It provides an opportunity to explore inner states that may appear as chaotic. During delirium the dying person is likely to be engaging with unfinished business, waging heroic battles, reviewing life, preparing for dying, and making spiritual connections. Those experiencing delirium appear to shift between worlds, working on the same issues from different aspects. Even though we may not be able to understand what those are, we attempt to follow the state and enter the reality that the person is in, helping them to unfold it and if possible, complete it. Believing in the state itself is very important. Joining the state through mirroring verbal expressions and physical behaviours can bring profound understanding.

With many delirium states the person may make sounds and move in ways that frighten or disturb us. It is important to be aware of our own edges to loud sounds and unpredictable movements. For example, a son says to his father who is dying: 'I love you, Dad". His father starts to yell something and the son in reaction, freaks out. From a process-oriented perspective the father's yelling is seen as positive feedback, as his response to his son's expression is a very energetic one. The father may be trying to express a big feeling too. We need to be familiar with our own altered states and sufficiently fluid to leave our consensus reality world behind and join the patient in their experience, trying to dream about and access the deeper meaning in the states they are experiencing. Once we understand more of what is trying to happen there, we can make it meaningful for the patient and then attempt to make a link between the patient's usual identity and the more secondary experience of the delirium.

I remember when Mike was experiencing a delirium, moving in and out of an altered state, he was giving orders to someone in a business-like manner while at the same time smiling. I knew he liked to manage people, but was always a bit shy about taking his power. Now he was being very precise, confidently giving orders and enjoying himself. I join him with the same precise manner and encourage him to keep enjoying what he is doing. He goes further, keeping an eye on the clock noting when it is 3 minutes past 12. He then says he has to go to the Post Office as someone wants him to sign some papers to sort something out. He continues to talk, nod his head and point his finger towards people I cannot see, saying he needs a programme. When he becomes lucid a short time later, he asks to be taken around the hospital in a wheel chair to say goodbye to the other patients and staff. This seems to be part of the programme he mentions earlier. I can tell that this experience is important to him. His dying provides him with an experience of power and authority that his everyday self was unable to fully achieve during his life.

In observing a delirium experience, we find it virtually impossible to make sense of what is happening. It is only when we join in the state ourselves, fully enter the experience and enact it too, that we begin to understand what it may be bringing for the person experiencing it. In supporting it and taking it further, it can be helping to complete "stuff" and bring to completion patterns that have cycled during life without resolution.

Dementia

In Praise of Craziness, of a Certain Kind[17]
On cold mornings
My grandmother,
With ownership of half her mind-
The other half having flown back to Bohemia-

Spread newspapers over the porch floor
So, she said, the garden ants could crawl beneath,
As under a blanket, and keep warm,

And what shall I wish for, for myself,
But, being so struck by the lightening of years,
To be like her with what is left, so loving.

Dementia is another altered state that brings us face to face with unknown and feared experiences. Dementia and its many forms, involves the gradual destruction of a

---

[17] Mary Oliver (in Shabahangi & Szymkiewicz, 2008)

person's memory, their ability to learn, reason, make judgments, communicate, and participate in everyday activities. It is estimated that 2 out of 3 people will have dementia in some form. Symptoms include seizures, falls, malnutrition, weight loss, frailty, visual impairment, sleep loss, oral disease, loss of control of emotions and inability to report pain. It is not surprising that we fear it and try to avoid it. In the West we place such store on a well-functioning mind that experiencing memory loss can bring stigma and shame.

We know through research and studies of the brain, that dementia affects parts of the brain associated with personality, behaviour and language. Abnormal proteins are deposited in the brain, destroying certain areas. Cells die leaving holes in the brain tissue, which then contracts. The most common types of dementia are Alzheimer's and Vascular Dementia resulting from small strokes (TIA's). From a biomedical view, dementia is a progressive and terminal illness. People are cared for either at home or, in the later stages, in a care facility. In palliative care, the focus is on making sure the person is comfortable and their dignity preserved.

Current attitudes and approaches to dementia can prevent us from viewing it as anything more than a disease. However, from a process-oriented view, Alzheimers and Dementia involve complex soulful and spiritual growth processes. Richards & Tomandl[18] have found that even in most advanced dementia cases, someone is always 'home' and is endeavouring to

---

[18] Richards & Tomandl (2010) *An Alzheimer's Surprise Party*

communicate with themselves and others as best they can. Using process-oriented skills they show how two-way communication and relationship is possible even in the most advanced dementia states. If we stay open, with a beginner's mind, curiosity, and respect for what is happening, then we will discover that although personality and behaviour do change, often dramatically, inherent character traits, beliefs, and memories can remain intact and offer doorways for communication.

As with other altered states found at end of life, we may not know a lot of what is happening on the inside, and this is the same for a person with advanced dementia. However, some or all of the following things could be happening:

• Completing unfinished business; meeting new or partially lived aspects of oneself
• Harvesting a life-time of experiences, making sense of and putting into perspective the process of life
• Making spiritual connections, deepening insight into relationship dilemmas, working with cultural and social conflicts.

From a Process Work perspective people with dementia are living at a dreaming level of consciousness. What is happening is not so much a problem to be solved but a dance between different worlds[19].

Being forgetful means that the person is opening to other aspects of themselves, other worlds. They are becoming free of consensus reality. This does not mean they are

---

[19] Shabahangi & Szymkiewicz (2008)

diminished as a person. They have changed. We need to change, too, in order to fluidly join them and support what is happening.

I visited a Residential Care Facility where the staff was running a day programme for people with Dementia. I was asked to sit with an elderly Indian man, I will call Peter, who was sitting in the corner not wanting to participate in any activities. Staff members were concerned about him because he had recently been told that his son had been killed in a motorbike accident. They were unsure as to whether he had taken this news in. He would not talk and showed no feelings.

I introduced myself and said I was just going to sit with him for a while if that was all right. He nodded. We sat together in silence for some time until one of the staff came by accompanying another patient to a room. The staff member had brown skin and may also have been from India. Peter suddenly pointed saying: "That is my son!" I commented on how wonderful it must be to have his son so close and then went further by asking him about his son, and their relationship. He responded in a slow measured way, telling me about how proud he was of him and how he loved him. Tears ran down his cheek. I reached out and held his hand and we sat in silence for a while. He then stood up and said he was ready to go back to the group.

Although we often cannot make sense of what the person with dementia is trying to express, and we find it difficult to understand the way their language is strung together and communicated, we can in any event put our way of understanding and being in consensus reality

78

aside, to enter the world and experience of that person, even though their reality may seem garbled to us. In the case above rather than saying that the staff member wasn't actually his son, I supported his dreaming process in seeing his son and by joining him as he unravelled his story. This allowed him to get in touch with his grief, which was very meaningful for him. Here is another case example to further illustrate.

Betty was 78 years old when it was noticed that she had become very distracted and somewhat agitated. She had a hard time focusing on communicating with others. She read every sign, number and street name that she saw while in the car, and often forgot the names of family members or who they were. As her dementia progressed she began to speak in French (the language of her childhood) and no longer seemed to hear or understand spoken English. She also began to pick at her skin and wring her hands a lot. Over time, the wounds on her hands and arms became severe and staff at the residential care facility were in a dilemma about how to deal with this. They did not feel right about restraining her hands but felt this was the only way in which they could curtail her from the repetitive picking of her own skin.

On my visit to her she was sitting up in a chair and gazing blankly around the room. She did not seem to register when I greeted her. She mumbled to herself in French, which I couldn't understand, and then became silent for some moments, her head and body sinking downwards as though she were collapsing in on herself.

She suddenly straightened up, made some high-pitched sounds and spoke a few foreign words, and then in a very agitated manner reached for her arm and began to pinch and pick at a scab. I pulled my chair very close to hers, put my face in her line of vision and made some sounds duplicating the pitch of the words she had spoken. I waved my hands around, copying the pace of her movements. I intensified the loudness, pitch and rhythm of the sounds I made, and grabbing hold of a pillow began to wrestle with it, pinching and clutching it. At the same time, I manoeuvred the pillow onto her lap, and sitting across from her guided her hands onto it, both of us plucking at the pillow. She really got into it, and as we continued together, her words became more distinguishable at first in French and then she began to utter some English words as well. After about 15 minutes the words became linked and formed a comprehensible sentence. "You will not do it ... you will not do it", she repeated over and over again in a cadence that began to sound like a song to me. I joined her in the song and then added a gesture, emphatically pointing and waggling my finger at a spot in the room, as if I was addressing a person there. She got very excited by this, sat up taller and also began to use her finger to point. A smile began to form on her face and her eyes brightened. As we continued, her smile became bigger and she looked overjoyed. She grabbed my hand and gave me a big squeeze then quietened down. After sitting with her for a short time, I noticed that she had fallen into a peaceful sleep. Staff reported to me on ensuing days, that she was much calmer and had stopped picking at herself.

From this example you will notice that I used a number of interventions to engage with Betty and to catch her attention. At no time did I attempt to pull her out of her state or get her to recognize everyday reality. I rather entered her experience by getting close to her, mirroring her in auditory, movement and relationship channels by duplicating her signals in my own expression. I then amplified her expression by enlarging it myself, making sounds more loudly than she, and movements bigger and stronger. In other words, I modelled for her what she was doing. In addition, I used my own dreaming to get in touch with what seemed to be a good direction for her in imagining that she was attempting to communicate something to someone with the same intensity as her voice and body movements. In seeing her pinching, I hypothesized that she needed to be more pinch-like in her interactions with others, and therefore introduced the accusatory finger that pinpointed the missing figure that she was addressing in her verbal expression. In seeing her positive feedback to this I knew I was on the right track and so we were able to unfold the process and bring it to a moment of resolution.

This is not a complicated intervention. It is based on signal and channel awareness of the other's expression and the ability to join with them in that. If nothing else, even if not unfolded fully, an intervention like this, no matter how small, helps the other feel supported and understood and can make a wealth of difference to their feeling experience.

In concluding this chapter, we would like to emphasize that using the skills mentioned above for working with people in altered states, allows us to share and enter another's perception of reality. We do this by joining and following their experience, bringing awareness in whatever way we can to what is happening there and supporting them to go further. The exercises in Part 2 will assist you in gaining insight into what it is like to be in a far-out state of consciousness, and will provide you with helpful tools and interventions to use with others.

Chapter 5

Metaphor, Dreams and Spirituality
Guidelines for the Mythical Journey

Each life is formed by its unique image -
an image that is the essence of that life and calls it to a
destiny.

- James Hillman

As mentioned previously, a person near death tends to move in and out of different states of consciousness. They may wake up and say something no one can understand. They are in their own realm at that moment. Our expectations of how things should be can lead us to dismiss or misinterpret such communication as it makes little sense to us. We may tend to intervene with the use of medication, or by talking concretely and directly to the person in an attempt to bring them back to this reality. However, if we listen carefully to what has been said we may notice that they are using symbolic language or metaphor to convey information to us. It is almost as if they are being carried by their mythical journey which is often mysterious to us and challenging to understand from our usual frame of reference.

There are a number of ways in which we can elicit and elaborate on mythical information from patients and family members.

- Personal and family stories
- Early childhood dreams and early memories
- Recurring patterns
- Passions and interests held during life
- Personal possessions – photographs – the way things are placed – absence of things – absence of family – family relationships
- Our own *dreaming* / intuition
- Synchronicities and signs in the environment
- Symbols, metaphors and dreams

Metaphor

We use metaphor many times a day. It is a figure of speech, a symbolic representation that we use to describe one kind of thing, or experience, by using another[20]. It implies a mirroring of one thing for another, both having common characteristics. For example, "she is a night owl." This tells us that she stays up at night like the owl. "That person has a cross to bear" meaning that the person feels burdened.

---

[20] Lakoff & Johnson (1980)

Metaphor is the language of dreams and dreamland experiences. When a person is dying they may detach from everyday life as it becomes less important to them. Instead they may appear to be focused in a different reality. They use metaphor as a way of letting us know what they encounter in their reality and, for example, when they might die; or what they need in order to die peacefully. One example of this would be the mention of a vehicle that is about to leave for another destination, often appearing in the metaphor of a ship about to set sail, or a train about to leave the station.

Research reveals that certain metaphors are commonly associated with dying[21]. Metaphors that tend to be present at death include the idea of being on a journey, packing bags, crossing bridges, getting to the airport, connecting with guides, navigating barriers or obstacles. When following a process, we view metaphors as entry points or dream doors to the patient's experience. We may try to interpret the metaphor, or make associations to it, but rather assist the person in discovering the meaning behind the metaphor through their experience of what is happening to them.

Although we can follow and amplify the outer experiences of the patient and believe they are a reflection of the dreamland and sentient experiences, we often don't know what is happening in their inner world; their internal visions, feelings, unfolding stories in the world they are in. As mentioned, it is helpful to know

---

[21] Bulkeley and Bulkley (2005)

something about their history and family dynamics to help with an understanding of what may be happening for them in the moment. We can also accompany and guide them, both by dreaming along with them and understanding the metaphors and the way they are being used.

I remember Mike, who was an avid collector of model fire engines. Some days before his death he looked up at his models and stated that there was still work to be done. Over the next days he went in and out of consciousness. One day he spoke from a dreamy state saying that the fire engine was packed all over the top and down the sides and there was a trailer as well and it was all ready to go. He died a few days later.

We can also use the patient's expression as metaphor for deeper experiences. We can sometimes pick up a little of this. For example, I remember a patient physically pulling her body back and crying when I came into the room. This patient had been inundated with visitors and practitioners of all kinds trying to help her through her vegetative state and back to the "real world". From this physically expressed metaphor, we can understand that she might need more of her own inner dreaming world and the sentient experiences in there. I remember withdrawing from the room with the comment that I would prefer her to have the space she needed to be with her own process. She immediately closed her eyes and withdrew into herself. We can take this as positive feedback to the intervention.

Here is an extract from a case study reported by a colleague who had visited a patient in his role as hospital chaplain.[22]

Fred was an 80 year-old Caucasian male, with CVA (cerebro-vascular accident/stroke). When I visited him the patient was no longer speaking much, mostly nodding. Two days after my visit, staff reported that Fred was actively dying and I made a follow-up visit. Jane, Fred's wife, made reference to his agitation & restlessness. We paused to observe in quiet. I held Fred's hand in mine and with my other hand, matched his breathing rhythm with a light touch.

Then Fred began doing a fascinating motion with his arm & hand, making small circular rotations "Jane, didn't you tell me Fred loved to fish," I asked. She responded, "oh, yea-ah. He even gave up his golf so he could fish." "By God, Jane, I think he's fishing," I said. "Hey, Fred, you fishin'?"

Fred began making verbalizations. Not sentences or even words. More like grunts, "Rrrmp, Ughh." I joined him "Rrrmph, Ughh" as together, I imagined us reeling in a fish. Continuing to dream into Fred's fishing experience, after more sounds and reeling movements, I offered, "I'm just wondering, God just might be reeling you in, bringing you home ... ya know ... one ... last ... run ..."

---

[22] Yamamoto, Dean – personal communication

More silence from Fred. No more reeling. Then Jane spoke. "Look at that! That's a smile." And with that Fred lay back and relaxed. The next morning, Jane told me that Fred was no longer agitated after our time together. The facility called at 1:00 a.m. the next morning to report Fred had died peacefully, moments before.

This illustration provides us with a wonderful example of how catching the deeper meaning of a metaphor, and taking it further through the process of amplification and use of our own dreaming, can bring resolution to some inner dilemma for the patient, allowing for completion of part of the patient's process. In this case, the patient was able to let go when he became aware that he was being reeled in by a higher power.

Otherworldly phenomena may also be apparent. Some of these may appear as apparitions existing in Bardo states encountered after death, as in the Tibetan Buddhist tradition; in vivid dreams; visions of ancestors; and other figures such as angels, spiritual guides, etc. There can also be unpredictable happenings, things we can't explain, such as a patient who had been in a confused state suddenly sitting up to say something with great clarity and certainty. What is going on in these states? We can view these phenomena as participating events in the on-going process of finding meaning within the dying process. This may involve making connection to a larger purpose, gaining insight into next steps or completing unfinished business, or for example, making peace with God.

Synchronicity

Synchronicity is a term used to describe events or experiences that have no apparent cause but are part of a unified field that gives rise to observation and experience. Many philosophers and thinkers at different periods of history have referred to an ultimate unity of all existence, which is outside of time and space, and which expresses itself through symbols representing pieces of the self that need recognition[23]. If synchronicities are noticed, they can alert us to phenomena that are part of the field, and the patient's process, waiting to be known more consciously. Synchronous events seem to happen a lot when people are close to dying. If they can be explored they bring forth relevant information regarding what lies within the patient's process and the way of being offered to the patient by the synchronicity. It is as if something else that is beyond our control is involved in and supporting the mythical journey.

One day as I was sitting with a patient near death, talking about what she thought heaven would be like, a beautiful butterfly landed on a plant nearby. The butterfly caught her attention and she exclaimed with joyous delight remembering a dream from the previous night of a room filled with butterflies all of brilliant colours. This is how she imagined heaven to be. We talked more about butterflies, what they meant to her and how she might also be like a butterfly in certain ways. In unfolding the experience of the butterfly by becoming it and dreaming into its essential experience, she used words such as calm, light, peaceful and free. In

---

[23] Storr, A. (1983). *The Essential Jung*

embracing these qualities, she felt relieved of the challenges of both life and death.

Being attuned to outside stimuli and the synchronous events that visit can be extremely supportive and helpful in following the direction indicated by both the patient's process and the synchronicity. It seems that not only can we rely on more obvious or subtle signals; we are also aided by the outside context in the way it presents itself through synchronicities. The *dreaming* behind what we know and observe is something that we can learn to trust as a guide too as it shows itself through these momentary synchronicities that visit us.

Dreams Near Death

Why work with dreams at end of life? Dreams are often marginalised in our Western culture where we mostly place little emphasis on the messages that our dreams bring for us. However, from earliest times dreams were seen as deeply meaningful, bringing messages from higher beings, guides, God, goddesses, or other deities. Indigenous cultures worldwide view dreams as shamanic or prophetic messages emerging out of mystic realms. Even in biblical times, information in dreams was regarded as vital to the survival of nations, and was used to guide leaders in battles and journeys to far off lands.

With the development of psychology early last century, and the work of Freud and Jung, dreams took on a greater significance for personal growth and development. From a psychological perspective night time dreams are viewed as symbolic representation of parts of ourselves we are not yet aware of or that have been repressed in everyday life. Dreams are viewed as gateways to the unconscious.

Jung also recognised dreams as having a universal or archetypal quality in that he noticed similar dream figures occurring across individuals and cultures. His study of childhood dreams revealed recurring patterns in dreams that make themselves known to us throughout our lives. These patterns, or life myth processes, seemed to be more prominent at times of transition throughout life and also during the dying process. They present to us the long-term processes that we meet many times in a lifetime and that we grapple with repeatedly at different times.

Viewing night-time dreams through a process-oriented lens illustrates doorways into dreamland and sentient experience. Dreams are viewed as waking us up to parts of ourselves that are less known or marginalised in everyday life, occurring on different levels of awareness. Dreams also show us how we can navigate these levels in order to go into the unknown to make it more conscious. For example, in their book *Near Death Dreams*[24], the authors relate the following:

Suzanne, an elderly lady, who was struggling with the final stages of her disease, had the following dream. She sees a candle lit on the windowsill of the hospital room and finds that it suddenly goes out. Fear and anxiety ensue as the darkness envelops her. Suddenly the candle

---

[24] Bulkeley and Bulkley (2005)

lights on the other side of the window, and she awakens.
That same day Suzanne died completely at peace.

Dreams can be seen to originate in a sentient realm of subtle, preverbal tendencies, or *Dreaming*. Dreamwork is a way of connecting to the *Dreaming*, the expression of the source that gives substance to manifest life. These tendencies reveal the essence of dream symbols or figures. One way of discovering the incentive of dreams is by diving deeply into the non-verbal, pre-cognitive, as yet un-manifest essence level of the dream, allowing that to generate a movement, image, song, poem or story from within its depths. (See exercise Part II – chapter 4). This deep exploration may then bring a quality, energy or style of being that can be integrated into the process in the moment. From this experience of the sentient realm we glean information that is needed in our everyday lives.

On the other hand, near death dreams are often experienced as having a metaphysical or transpersonal quality. When we experience this type of dream we may find too that it speaks for itself and does not warrant any interpretation or analysis. The dream itself speaks so powerfully that the dreamer's response may be wonder and awe.

I once visited a woman, whom I will call Beth, who was struggling with her progressing cancer tumours, knowing she had only a short while to live. She was afraid of dying and had fallen into a deep depression at the thought of leaving her family. Beth believed that death was the end, that there was nothing after this life. During my visit I asked her about her family and what it was that particularly troubled her about leaving her family. As she talked she remembered a dream she had had that morning.

I am walking down a road with my husband, my son and daughter. The road ahead is in darkness. As we walk together my two children step back and my husband and I keep going together. I notice that he has a lantern. He hands me the lantern and steps back and I go on alone.

Beth began to cry, overcome by feelings of grief. She soon dropped into an exhausted sleep. I knew this dream had deep significance for her and for what was ahead of her. I came back later that day to find that she had gone out for a coffee with her son. She was feeling much better and was talking about the things she still needed to do. I asked her about her feeling response to the dream. She said it was when her husband gave her the lantern that she knew she would be alright. To her it represented the love they felt for each other that was now guiding her forward and would be with her forever. As she spoke about love I noticed her voice became softer and quieter, her face lit up and she smiled. I encouraged her to really feel what she was experiencing then. She nodded, closed her eyes, going inside, and became silent for a few moments. I was touched by the feeling sense of love that emanated from her. Beth told me later that she had not really acknowledged how deep that love was until then. She said she was no longer afraid of dying. She went home and had several more weeks of special time with her family.

Research supports dreams near death as having a metaphysical or spiritual quality that cannot be analysed[25]. In her research in which she collected 2500 dreams of people near death, Marie Louise von Franz, a Jungian Analyst, found dreams where "one feels compelled to leave them in space as a symbolic statement about another reality." Such dreams included those in which dead people visited the dying person. The dreams had a numinous quality and remained fresh for the person over long periods of time. This was evident in Beth's dream above. The profound love she felt stayed with her until her death some months later. Von Franz's research revealed that almost all symbols appearing in near death dreams are archetypal and are mirrored in various religious beliefs about life after death. The symbols are also evident as part of the individuation process, particularly in the second half of life[26]. Von Franz also reported that all the dreams of people facing death indicate the unconscious preparing the conscious mind not for an end, but for a profound transformation and a kind of continuation of the life process.

In a recent research study exploring the dreams of patients in Palliative Care[27], it was reported that dreams are a reflection of waking concerns that the dying are unable to speak about. These include concerns about illness, unresolved conflicts with significant others, and issues relating to impending death. The author's findings suggest that concerns about oneself, and others, tend to be reflected in dreams of palliative care patients across

---

[25] von Franz 1984 p. 157
[26] Ibid
[27] Sandu Iordache (2012)

gender, culture and other levels. He found that when patients talked about their dreams and made personal interpretations, information was revealed that was significant in providing appropriate care and support.

Spirituality at End of Life

Consideration of spirituality in hospice and palliative care, is acknowledged as being of central importance in attending to the dying. The holistic model of the hospice movement and palliative care endeavours to incorporate all dimensions of life into patient and family care. There is a growing demand to attend to a patient's spiritual needs at the end of life. However, at least in the West, we seem to struggle to incorporate a broader concept of spirituality that exists outside of formalized religion, and therefore have trouble recognizing, making sense of, and assisting patients who are experiencing spiritual phenomena.

Spirituality in the above context refers to an awareness of our deepest Self. It is the feeling sense of the creative force that imbues everything and lies behind all that is. Spirituality is also concerned with our connection to God, Tao, Chi, to nature, to essence, the Dreamtime, the Divine or transcendent. It is also a deep feeling sense of being pulled or guided by something bigger than oneself that gives meaning and purpose to our lives and deaths.

Spirituality for some is expressed through religion which is an established system of traditions, creeds, beliefs and practices commonly held by a particular group or community. Some of the world's major religions are Christianity, Hinduism, Islam, Judaism and Buddhism.

Each religion provides a set of rules and guidelines which members follow in order to build a relationship with God or Divine other. In recent times, with the influence of the East, indigenous cultures, quantum physics and a more personal search for an internal life, religion as we understand it is changing. We find ourselves faced with diverse views and experiences about the nature of reality and consciousness. This is particularly relevant when facing death and addressing questions about what happens when we die.

For those who are dying and their families, questions may arise relating to the meaning of life, identity, the reason why this is happening and what happens next. They may struggle to make meaning of what is happening and search for answers within spiritual, religious and cultural perspectives. Research reveals that spiritual beliefs and practices do assist people in coping with advancing disease and the process of dying.

Spiritual connectedness can occur in a number of ways, including re-connecting with beliefs and practices from childhood, or seeing visions of those who have died before us, or of our ancestors. There may also be experiences of psychic phenomena such as seeing angels, hearing music or voices, or experiencing one's body as dissolving or becoming ether. Spirituality is embedded in experience. Spiritual experience takes us beyond consensus reality into a state that is outside linear time and space. It is here that we have experiences that are fleeting, have a numinous quality, cannot be localised and are difficult to talk about.

In the West we tend to minimise or dismiss spiritual phenomena around dying, such as visions, viewing them as part of advanced disease and the dying brain.

If we don't make the mistake of assuming they (the dying) are confused, we are likely to feel some of the excitement they (visions) convey – for we are witnessing the momentary merging of two worlds that at all other times remain tightly compartmentalised and mutually inaccessible. The emerging is what I call the spirituality of dying[28].

If we view experience as coming out of the *dreaming* or sentient realm, made up of tendencies and pre-verbal signals, we can assist those near death both in believing in their deep experiences as well as in meeting and navigating them. The everyday self often struggles with the more unknown aspects of essence not having encountered it consciously before and it is here that we can be helpful. In some people, fear comes up during this stage with a tendency to resist the experiences that visit them. However, if there is an openness to these, many find deep joy and peace or an illumination of the future path.

I am thinking of Clare, a woman who was in the final hours of her life. She was a devout Christian and looking forward to "going to be with Jesus." From a drowsy state she told me that even though she was not afraid to die she was feeling scared of what was happening to her in the moment. She said she felt like she was "melting",

---

[28] Betty (2006, p.37).

that the part of her she identified with was slowly slipping away. I noticed that her out-breath was longer than her in-breath. Thinking that the melting experience was somehow important for her I asked if it would be okay if I supported her to melt even more. I told her that I would stay with her and melt with her. I told her that I would hold her hand and gently pace her breath to let her know I would be with her. She smiled and nodded confirming that it was the way to go. We noticed that on amplifying her out-breath she was able to get deeper into the melting experience. After a short while of my encouraging her to go deeper into melting she let out a sigh saying "Oh it is so beautiful! Yes, Jesus!" A tear rolled down her cheek. Those were her last words. She died peacefully that evening. I was deeply touched by this experience. There was something ecstatic about melting that took me momentarily into an experience of fluidity, a feeling sense of having no limits. I wondered if that was something of her experience, too. The atmosphere in the room was calm, light and peaceful. After she died I noticed she was smiling slightly as if she had discovered something delicious.

The mythical journey, something of which we have described above, offers us a doorway into the mysterious, numinous aspects of a person's path both through life and during death. Some believe that it is this thread that carries a being further into the next steps beyond death. It is at the end of life that we seem to once again meet long-term patterns related to the mythical journey of our unfolding lives. This pulls us to connect with the deepest aspects of who we are and what lies ahead.

In this chapter we have illustrated various ways in which to support this process through understanding the usefulness of metaphor, dreams and essence-like experiences. We have also suggested ways in which to use this awareness with patients. The tools offered here provide support for the dying process through the use of our own awareness in assisting the patient on his or her journey through the mysterious passage of death.

Chapter 6

Pain – The Ultimate Disturber

The wound is the place where the light enters you
                                                    - Rumi

Physical pain for those at end of life may be brought on by the progression of an illness, the effects of aggressive treatments and/or increasing discomfort as the body struggles to adapt to changes associated with the dying process. Severe pain is usually treated with medications. Some patients may choose to use alternative treatments such as acupuncture or herbal treatments, and pain management techniques including various meditations and visualizations. Pain may also be associated with psychological, relationship or spiritual disturbances, and in this way may be viewed as emotional or psychic pain. This kind of pain is frequently not recognized or spoken about, but when it is noticed and shared with others, some relief may occur.

Pain is something many of us fear. It is generally something we try to avoid or rid ourselves of. We often feel victimized by it and struggle to regain some control. We go into battle and fight it, attempt to resist it, generally tense up around it, and wish it were gone. Having chronic or severe pain is hard to live with and the more intense, the more tragic it seems to be. Many people say to me that they are not afraid of dying but the possibility of dying in unbearable pain is terrifying.

We know that our reactions to physical pain, such as dread, fear, tension and anxiety, tend to make it worse. Stephen and Ondrea Levine[29] observe how we tighten around pain both mentally and physically. They describe how our thinking about pain, illness and death can increase resistance to the pain, and how it can be exacerbated by those around us who are unable to recognize the extent to which it affects us. There are existing ways to work with reactions or resistance to pain through exercises to "manage" the pain, breathing techniques, visualizations, etc. Generally, most hospitals have pain clinics that support people with chronic pain issues. How we approach our own and other's pain near death has implications for care. For example, in the attempt to manage pain, sedating someone who would like to remain alert, can increase agitation and anguish.

Palliative Care focuses on the idea of total pain. This is an inclusive view of the experience of pain that incorporates the physical, emotional, social, existential and spiritual dimensions of our lives. Emotional pain

---

[29] Levine, Stephen and Ondrea (1982). *Who Dies?*

shows itself in states of depression, anxiety, fear, loneliness, anger, aggression, or resentment. Social or relationship pain has to do with disturbances in relationship that aren't addressed, or old relationship challenges that are incomplete and plague us. Existential and spiritual pain can be related to meaning, as in, "What is the meaning of what I am going through"? "Why me"? When no answers are found to these questions, existential suffering can increase.

Experiencing ongoing or acute pain is very disturbing and can challenge a person in their belief that they are able to cope. It is generally very difficult to find restfulness and ease when in the grip of pain. As mentioned, most of us tend to resist and try to ignore it, hoping it will go away. From a process-oriented perspective though, disturbance, in whatever form it presents to us, can be a great teacher if we are able to unravel an underlying message or meaning for our lives (or deaths). Within pain can be found a source of wisdom for our own growth of awareness, as well as an opportunity to integrate new qualities and aspects of ourselves, thus enriching our relationship to ourselves, to others, and our lives in general.

Rather than focusing on reactions to pain and attempting to control the pain itself, pain is viewed as a doorway into the person's dreaming process. In other words, what is held in the experience of pain, i.e. its nature, core energy or quality, can be something that the patient needs to integrate more in their awareness and their own repertoire of behaviour. While supporting the person's process in trying to fight it, we remain open to the meaning of what lies within it. We attempt to unfold the experience of pain just as we have described unravelling a process in previous chapters. It can be challenging to amplify an experience of pain, as initially it means enlarging it or feeling it more. However, once through that first step, one is able to go deeper into the channel experiences, transforming the pain itself into specific energies, figures or roles representing parts of oneself that may be marginalized. Getting to know more about these, and bringing them closer to everyday awareness, can help to reduce the pain experience. Please do remember that those in pain are usually extra-sensitive to stimuli. When approaching them, and especially when using touch, take care to check with them if what you are doing is okay. If they are unable to respond verbally ask them to give you a sign, and also watch carefully for feedback. You might also check in with medical staff as to any areas of the body that may be especially sensitive.

Morin and Reiss[30] describe their holistic approach in working with constant pain. They mention their work with a woman diagnosed with fibromyalgia. They were able to explore points of pain in her body that were particularly disturbing to her. They discovered that each point of pain contained not only discomfort, but also extraordinary memories and dream-like experiences connected to her personal history. Exploring and processing each of these points, helped her to express the underlying pain of her personal history and freed her to become more aware of information lying below the level of awareness. Grappling with these memories,

---

[30] Morin, P. & Reiss, G. (2010). *Inside Coma*

expressing her pain about these, and learning more about the underlying direction these symptoms pointed to, helped her to gradually become free of the worst of her physical pain.

Arnold Mindell[31] suggests that one reason we don't do well with pain is that we don't know or love our body's feelings. He suggests it is the lack of relationship to our bodies that makes us hesitant or shy about working with what is happening there. He says it is important to accept pain, to sit with it and feel it rather than attempt to get rid of it as fast as possible. He goes on to talk about a patient he worked with who was dying of stomach cancer.

He was lying in a hospital bed groaning and moaning in pain. Once when he was able to speak, he told me that the tumour in his stomach was unbearably painful. As he had already had a lot of operations I suggested trying a new approach, which the man was willing to do. I suggested making the pain even worse. He said he knew exactly how to do that and told me that the pain felt like something in his stomach trying to break out. If he helped it break out, he said the pain worsened. He lay on his back and started to increase the pressure in his stomach. He pushed his stomach out and kept pushing and pressing and exaggerating the pain until he felt as if he were going to explode. Suddenly at the height of his pain, he shouted out, "Oh Arny, I just want to explode, I've never been able to really explode!" At that point he switched out of his body experience and began to talk to

---

[31] Mindell, 1984, p.7

me. He told me that he needed to explode and asked if I would help him do so. "My problem," he said, "is that I have never expressed myself sufficiently, and even when I do, it's never enough".

The man's symptoms improved as Arny continued to see him and assist him with his process of 'exploding'. He finally died after two to three years, having learned to express himself better.

Making the pain worse may seem unusual, even crazy. Generally, we tend to avoid as much as possible going into feeling the pain as we want it to go away, and hence we resist it. Patients too will not generally be willing to enter their experience of pain until we explain to them the purpose in doing so. Let's remember that disturbance, when explored and unfolded, often becomes an ally to us in offering something useful to us such as a particular quality or energy, which is held in the nature of the pain experienced. In this story we see how staying with the pain and amplifying it brings relief and something new. The patient gained insight into how important it was to him to express himself more fully and not to hold back.

Approaching pain as a signal or doorway into the dreaming process means we can work with it in a number of ways. We can:

• Amplify the pain by getting sensory-grounded information about it and extend the experience of it into other channels.

- Create a figure out of the channel experiences and imagine being that figure in order to find its useful energy.
- Become the pain-maker. In other words, expressing the kind of force or energy that would create that kind of pain. In this way we discover whether we need the energy of the pain-maker more ourselves, or whether it has an agenda or teaching that will expand our awareness of our own nature.
- Use drawing to depict it. In looking at the drawing we may get a sense of what it is trying to represent for us. Something from the drawing may catch our attention and we can take this further in another drawing or represent it in other channels to round out the experience of it.
- Go into the essence of the pain experience to find its pre-manifest tendency.
- Use song and movement to work with the disturbance and the person's reaction to it.

For example, as I sit here writing, I notice I have a small ache in the base of my neck that spreads out to my shoulders. Using sensory-grounded information I would describe it as dull, constant and hard like a board. Now I start to amplify it using the feeling of hardness. I begin to harden other parts of my body more and more. As I do that and intensify it, I notice that I become stiff and hard all over my body. I feel immovable. I know I could use this in my writing right now as I have so many ideas coming and going which serve to distract me from my own thoughts. I could certainly use more of that immovability in my daily interactions, too, as I tend to be rather malleable and sometimes even compliant. I have a hard time standing up for my position or experience. I might take the experience of being the hard board even further to discover its essence or pre-manifest tendency. To do this I go inside myself bringing my attention to the quality or essence of the board, its hardness. With curiosity and an open mind, I explore what gave rise to it. What was there before it became hard, it's original tendency? As I go deeper into it, I discover an experience of being "here", fully present and solid, nothing else on my mind, holding firmly. I make a small hand movement that expresses what I am feeling and the word "focus" pops up. I am encouraged by this experience and know that by bringing more focused attention to what I am doing in the moment I will be able to go further in my work and relationships.

Alternatively, instead of using sensory-grounded information to access the experience, I could draw the image I am having of the board. In gazing at the drawing, I might notice something that stands out for me there. I can explore that further by drawing that part of it on its own, amplify the shape and colour in my new drawing and then use movement and sound to bring that out further. As I do that, I notice the emphasis I give to drawing the board and its straight lines. The lines become more emphatic and focused as I add to the drawing – more solid and entrenched. This is the same immovability and focus that I arrived at through the other method I used described above.

Here is a further example described by a young woman suffering for many years from migraines[32].

Eventually, I discovered there was neither anything physically wrong with me causing the migraines, nor was there anything that could eliminate the pain completely. And strangely, no prophylactics worked. By this time my symptom was severely restricting my ability to live and having an enormous impact on my family, emotionally and financially. During this time my general health had also deteriorated. My doctor began to talk of a pain syndrome and that I would benefit from being on anti-depressants. This effectively made me feel neurotic, overly sensitive and somehow at fault, alone and different from 'normal' people. With 3-4 days of every week spent struggling with pain as well as being wiped-out by migraine medication, I finally realised I needed to seek a wider frame.

In the midst of this despair, I was introduced to a Process Work therapist who suggested that there may be something 'right' about my symptom, not something wrong with me; that my symptom may well hold meaning for my life and not only be a cause of great suffering. It was explained that there can be important information in our symptoms which needs to come to our attention and find expression and, (more bizarrely to me) that the symptom could contain the seeds of its own solution. I focused on where the migraine pain initially appeared - an intense, throbbing ache in my temples. I noticed there was warmth which gradually increased as I brought my

---

[32] Scott, L. (2014). *Out of the Matrix* (unpublished manuscript)

attention to it, until my entire head began to feel hot and pulsating. I then had an image of a planet throbbing, overheating, a huge fiery ball of energy about to explode. Encouraged to let what wanted to happen, happen, I imagined it exploding.

I saw the entire planet shatter and shoot pieces far out into the atmosphere, scattering everywhere. As I described what I 'saw', my hands were also exploding outward. I was encouraged to stand up and allow my entire body to feel this enormous amount of energy sending bits of itself into space in great arcs. As this planet, I experienced an amazing sensation of having colossal energy and power. Surprisingly, I found myself laughing, unusually buoyant and completely energised by this incomprehensible process.

Pain may also be linked with cultural and social issues, reflecting biases, marginalization, or polarizations within that culture or social setting. In a group setting, colleagues Pierre Morin[33] and Jai Tomlin work with Vivian, a woman who suffers from severe headaches. She describes her headaches as really painful and on the right side of her head where it gets really tense. Her left side is usually relaxed. The pain keeps her awake at night. The symptom had begun a year prior after a very stressful time. She describes how her right side becomes numb, the intense pain lasting about 15 minutes. In one instance she felt dizzy for 2 hours and went to the hospital for a check-up and tests. Vivian lives in Greece where she says there is a lot of tension in the

---

[33] Morin, P. (2015). *Health in Sickness, Sickness in Health*

atmosphere. She reports having relationship problems at the time the headache started.

In order to get a sense of how Vivian experiences the headache, Pierre and Jai ask her to show them how to create the pain using a cushion. Vivian begins to twist the cushion and when encouraged to amplify it she makes strong squeezing, twisting and drilling motions and starts to growl. Pierre and Jai support her to go further. After some hesitation Vivian's growl becomes a powerful "No, I am not going to sit on the couch!" She then unfolds the conflict between the part of her that wants to relax (sit on the couch) and the part that just wants to go all out and make the most of her life. She feels held back by consensus reality conventions. As the process unfolds further through role-play Vivian gets to know more about the two sides, the one that wants to rest and the one that wants to be active. She becomes aware of how she needs both and talks about how she can befriend both and have them relate to each other.

Pierre then asks about how this awareness could be applied in Greece when she goes home. She says:

"The first thing that comes to mind is how amongst my community in Greece we tend to blame each other for not doing what each of us thinks is best. Not out there enough. Many people can go out on the streets and other people need to stay and care, need to garden. Doing different things. We don't appreciate the diversity, thinking we all have to do the same thing in the same way".

Interesting to notice too, that at present Greece has been criticized by the rest of the world for being "lazy" and not using enough energy to make things work in the country, while some in Greece are upset by this, protesting how hard they work in order to survive there. We can therefore see that Vivian's process pretty much mirrors the polarity in the larger field in which she lives. Her struggle between opposing parts may well be a reflection of the different roles present in her social context. In the next chapter we will go further into field theory and illustrate how the individual is closely connected to other levels in society, namely on the relationship and systemic levels, and how we might choose to address these.

In the above chapter we have described a few of the interesting ways to explore the dreaming found within experiences of pain. You might like to try for yourself using the exercises on working with pain in Part II.

Chapter 7

Interventions in Relationships, Families, Systems

The quest for wisdom is rooted in an erotic relationship to the world – a deep desire to know love and passion before one dies

- Cornel West

Dying is not just about the individual patient, but also about those around them and the environment in which they find themselves. As someone who may be part of the care team, or working more personally with the patient's process, we may observe or be called on to mediate/facilitate interactions between patients and their families or family members, or between patients and staff. We may also need to navigate the style, rules and structures of the system itself, which in some cases we may perceive as limiting our opportunity to engage and support the patient.

There are many different process-oriented tools and techniques that support us to engage with dynamics such as the above. These have developed from the foundations of field theory[34] and deep democracy[35].

Deep democracy refers to the value that all parts hold within the whole. We tend to value certain parts over others, have preferences towards one or the other, and avoid or marginalize those that have "negative" connotations in our eyes or in the eyes of the culture in which we live. However, if we are to be able to truly support emerging process we need to be prepared to give all aspects an opportunity to express themselves and be supported by us.

Field theory explores how roles within a particular context coexist and reflect each other. The state of any part or position in a field is dependent on every other part or position found within that same field. The field is a dynamic representation of all that is within it, in which parts entangle, interconnect and mirror each other in some way. The family or systemic field is a fluid, evolving background pattern that contains and is created by everything that it surrounds.

The field can be felt; it is hostile or loving, repressed or fluid. It consists not only of such overt, visible, tangible structures as meeting agendas, party platforms and rational debate, but also hidden, invisible, intangible

---

[34] Lewin, Kurt (1943). Defining the "Field at a Given Time." *Psychological Review.*
[35] Mindell, A. (1995) *Sitting in the Fire*

emotional processes, such as jealousy, prejudice, hurt and anger[36].

Every field has its particular atmosphere, its disturbing elements, its unrecognized aspects, as well as the various influences it exerts on all within it. An individual's experience within a particular field is often also part of others' experience in the same field, even though that part may not be consciously recognized. Parts in the field may align with each other, or they may be polarized against each other, holding different positions or views.

Let's try to make this quantum idea more practical through an example.

The sister of a patient who had been in a deep coma for more than 4 months, called me in to consult about whether to continue to keep the patient on life support. Other members of the family were now at a point where they were insisting that keeping the patient alive was creating suffering for her. Doctors had given a poor prognosis and did not foresee the patient coming out of the comatose state. The facility where the patient was being cared for was also becoming impatient, requesting that the patient be moved to another facility for long-term care as they were in need of the extra bed. However, my client (the patient's sister – Anne) was convinced that the patient wanted to live and could not contemplate ending her life.

In looking at this situation from a field perspective, we can see that the field is somewhat polarized. Anne wants

---

[36] Mindell, A. (1995) *Sitting in the Fire.* P. 19

her sister to continue on life support, believing this is what her sister would want. Other family members think it is time to withdraw support and end the suffering. From the facility's point of view, the bed is needed for other patients. Staying or leaving is the central conflict between the positions occupied by members of the field.

I visited the patient (Betty) on a number of occasions and was able to create a binary mode of communication with her. I had noticed that her right eyelid periodically blinked and in working with her, was able to bring the signal to her awareness. I encouraged her to use the blink as a "yes" to questions I asked her. We tried this out and practiced it over a number of visits until her "yes" responses were consistent. (When there was a "no" present for her in response to my questions she did not give the signal). Then we were finally ready to negotiate the big question, "do you want to continue with life support"? I asked this of her a number of times, and her answer was consistently "yes". As I was putting this question to her for the last time, Anne burst excitedly into the room. "I have just received confirmation that such-and-such Care Facility has a bed available and will welcome Betty. The field appeared to be supporting the patient's decision to live on and had provided a home for her.

Fields are created in part by the interaction between roles and ghost roles (roles that are not identified or expressed in interaction but are implied, felt and part of the background atmosphere). In the example above, those wanting to take Betty off life support were in the majority and exerted a lot of influence. This role might be seen as an authority role, occupied by those who thought they knew what was best for the patient. On the other side, in another role in the field was Anne, who was unsure of the best thing to do, appearing uncertain and hesitant. As Betty was not able to verbalize, her position was unknown. The missing voice from the patient is a ghost in the field, while holding a lot of central focus and power over the family. Another ghost role was the one who could welcome and support the patient unreservedly. This role appeared at the very same moment that it became clear that Betty wanted to live, reinforcing the decision to continue with life support as the correct one.

It is often the interaction between the roles that brings clarity or insight. All organizations / groups / families have roles they more readily identify with such as: family head; president; administrator; youngest son, most successful; more intelligent, etc. These are more consensus reality based positions. Other roles like oppressor; dictator; listener; disturber; elder; supporter, etc. are not so readily identified with, as these are less familiar or known than the more primary roles. They are aspects of Dreamland. It is usually very helpful to the field and those within it, to identify and name the lesser known and the ghost roles, and in some cases to step into those roles and speak for them, representing them for the field.

Dreamland roles are not usually taken into consideration in interaction. As we are mostly unaware of these, we do not consciously identify with them. However, bringing them out in dialogue and negotiation can be very helpful to the field, as that will support the deepening of the interaction and bring more awareness to what lies beneath more apparent and recognizable experience. It also helps to give more insight into the best ways to deal with challenge or conflict. When we participate in the field as therapists, caregivers, family supporters, practitioners, and so on, it is helpful to keep awareness of what roles are present and how they interact with each other. We are then in a position to support the field's interaction and further development by drawing attention to these aspects of relationship and the various positions that are held. Metacommunication (see chapter 3) is probably the most useful tool we can use at these times. It is unbiased, neutral, and frames the situation for the group, bringing awareness to what lies beneath the surface of interaction. Metacommunicating about atmospheres, feelings, places of tension, unacknowledged reactions, and changes in expression, can be very helpful in assisting those present to recognize dynamics that may usually go unnoticed. This can be enlightening to those who are present and can help to resolve difficulties.

In addition to being *awake* to field dynamics concerning the family, sometimes we are called on to also negotiate with the larger system within which the patient is living. Systems and organizations generate their own field dynamics and in supporting the patient, we find ourselves needing to adhere to the rules and styles of interacting within the system itself. In addition, we come face-to-face with the belief systems functioning there.

When in interaction with members who represent the system, particularly if we find ourselves either polarized against the system, or caught in a conflict between the patient and/or the patient's family and the system itself, it is useful to harness one's awareness and notice what the atmosphere is like there, what roles are present (as well as ghost roles), etc., and to try to metacommunicate about what is noticed in an objective way. As we mention above, this also supports more awareness for others and a potential to go deeper in interaction and get more insight into what is attempting to happen in that field. Here is an example.

I was called in to visit a patient who had been in an accident and who had suffered considerable brain damage. He was in a coma, but did seem to react to my presence by moving his eyes around to look at me. His good friend wanted me to assess the patient and give my opinion about his state as well as visit him on an ongoing basis in order to work with his process.

On my third visit there, I brought in my video camera as I wanted to video my work with the patient in order to study it when alone. I had received written permission from the friend, who was acting as his next of kin. However, the nurse reacted strongly to this, "reporting" me to the head nurse and chief administrator. We met together to discuss the situation further.

I experienced a lot of pressure from both parties to relinquish my position and let go of the camera. They held powerful roles in that field, and I had very little influence there.

After some back and forth arguing, mostly about the ethics of the situation and the impropriety of what I was doing, I noticed that whenever I mentioned using the recording for research and further learning, there was a pause in which tension relaxed a little and the others looked over at me as if wanting to know more. I brought this to their awareness, metacommunicating about what I perceived as their interest in research and learning. This comment opened up a new avenue of conversation about research and development that brought us closer together. My intervention defused the situation. The atmosphere changed and we went on to have a meaningful conversation, which resolved our conflict. They agreed to allow me to videotape the patient with a signed statement from me agreeing to their terms.

My example above may appear to some readers as being too challenging to negotiate, or beyond their skills. However, intervention can be made just by verbally describing what you notice in the field, no matter how small. You will surprise yourself at how effective you can be.

Relationships

Another level of the field reflecting field dynamics is that which occurs in relationship interaction. As many of us are aware, the death process brings to the fore relationship dynamics that have remained unaddressed. Death itself seems to confront us with unfinished relationship "stuff" as people prepare to leave. Perhaps it is in the nature of completion that we are faced with these.

We can notice signals in the patient's behaviour to others that alert us to underlying issues between the patient and those in contact with him/her. These come up toward specific family members, or to staff; in the relationship between family members themselves; between the patient or family member and the system representative. For some of us working closely in this situation it is useful to have some handy tools in order to bring awareness to what is happening and to help the relationship along a little. These skills are also extremely useful for us in our own relationships in everyday life.

There are many aspects to relationship that we can focus on, and a whole array of process-oriented skills at our disposal. For the purpose of processing the situations you may find yourselves in, we are introducing some main concepts illustrated by matching exercises that you will find in Part II.

Relationship Styles

Some styles in relating are marginalized by cultural, social and personal expectations. We usually operate in terms of our primary style (culturally and internally approved style), while other styles are less favoured. It can be helpful to adopt another style as this helps to bring in another part of oneself to the conversation and can also help the other to feel acknowledged for his or her own particular style. Try it out with a friend. Relate in your usual style for a couple of minutes, and then switch to a style that you may have admired in someone else or a style you find disturbing. Notice what difference, if any, occurs in your interaction with your friend.

When we are relating to others we can sometimes notice an expression, tone of voice, movement, or posture that stands out or doesn't seem to quite go along with the other's style. These signals are gateways into another aspect of this person that has a different style or way of expressing/being. Noticing these can help you deepen the interaction by supporting the more secondary style and inviting it in. Here is an example.

I remember a rather irate nurse who was very irritated by the husband of her patient. The patient was in a deep coma, and had been for five years. The husband, believing that she was not getting sufficient nourishment, would bring in specially enriched liquids to put in the patient's feeding tube. Of course, the nurse was aghast at this and upset by the husband's persistence in doing so. Her tone toward him was usually tinged with anger and resentment. One day, the patient's husband was looking particularly drawn and fatigued. The nurse was in the room (I was there, too) when he arrived to visit his wife and greeted him in her usual surly way. However, I noticed that before turning away to attend to the patient, she glanced at him with a concerned expression on her face. At the same time, her voice softened as she addressed him. I pointed out to the nurse, that she looked touched by something she had noticed in the husband. She responded that she was worried about him because he looked so drained. "After all", she said, "he is like an old friend in some ways. I have been seeing him nearly every day for some years now ... and besides ... I would worry about my patient if he wasn't here for her". On saying that, she turned toward the husband and reached out to touch his hand. He was overjoyed.

So we can see, how pointing out a relationship signal, even though it may be subtle, can both change the relationship between two people and also bring something new into the field.

Moods

Why is it important to notice moods? We generally fluctuate in our moods on a more or less daily basis. However, when faced with major change or in a critical situation, our emotions and feeling expressions may be stronger or more volatile than usual. Moods of various sorts are often noticed in the patient's room and context. These may arise in the patient him/herself or in family and staff members. There are many ways to address a mood that may be present, but we would like to focus on one way of addressing a mood that is useful in the context of the dying experience. That is the concept of high and low dreams.[37]

When in relationship with someone else, it is likely that we have certain expectations and hopes for the relationship. We often spend many years longing for a vision or ideal that we can't quite grasp, or that doesn't come our way. This is the high dream. A patient, who expects and hopes that her family will be attentive when she is ill, is in a high dream of what she would like the relationship to bring. Often the high dream state is full of energy, positivity and wellbeing.

---

[37] Mindell, Arnold (1995). *Sitting in the Fire*

However, if the high dream does not eventuate, if our hopes and longings do not come true, then we are often catapulted out of the uplifted state into a low dream experience. This may produce sadness, loss, depression, anger or hopelessness.

It can be very useful to notice the moods present and to help with awareness of them by framing what you notice in terms of the feeling aspects, e.g. disappointment, excitement, and so on. If the patient or family member appears angry or depressed it is likely that a high dream has not eventuated for them. It can be transformative to make mention of the mood you notice in the room, and then to unfold these further together with the patient, family or staff, in order to trace the underlying, unnoticed experiences present. This often leads to a deep sharing of previously unrecognized and unexpressed thoughts and feelings bringing people closer together. A simple statement such as, *"I'm feeling some tension in the room"*, or *"this must be a sad moment for you"* when you're feeling a certain atmosphere in the room, and then an invitation to talk further about it, can help to relieve relationships by bringing out the unsaid experiences that people are holding.

Rank Issues

Everyone has both more and less rank than someone else. Rank implies power difference.[38] There are different aspects to rank that we generally do not recognize. We may have social rank in terms of social aspects such as whether we're employed or not, and if we are in what

---

[38] Mindell, Arnold (1995, p. 58). *Sitting in the Fire*

sectors; our physical appearance; our economic standing; our skin colour; sexual orientation, etc. We may have psychological rank in that we have more awareness than others as to what is going on in terms of interpersonal dynamics in any given moment, or we may have more spiritual rank in feeling more comfortable or detached in challenging situations. Unconscious rank creates trouble in relationship as it leaks out without awareness and tends to cause escalations or reactions in others. What we mean by rank unconsciousness is:

- Rank is personal privilege. When unconscious, the person does not recognize or identify the privileges they have in certain contexts. For those with less privilege, this may be inflammatory as the discrepancy goes unnoticed by the person with rank who is unaware of what their privilege brings for them.
- The use of one's authority and power without being aware that the other may feel oppressed by that. In other words, I would not be using my power well if those with whom I'm in relationship, feel put down, marginalized or diminished in some way.
- When possessing social rank in terms of one's economic position, physical ability, age, etc. and with little awareness of how comfortable it is to identify with that. Not realizing that others may not have those attributes or be as comfortable as I am in those same areas.

When people are unaware of their rank and the position that gives them, others around them tend to react in a variety of ways ranging from feeling insecure or "less than" to escalating or becoming resentful. This can lead to compliance, outright conflict, rebellion, stalemates or a process of revenge or sabotage. We can notice some of these dynamics in the family interactions that happen either with or around the patient.

As an observer, we might wish that we had the skills or tools to help in these situations. When you notice a discrepancy in rank and the relationship between people suffering as a result, please do summon up your courage to bring awareness to what is happening. If you can do this without blame or judgement, those receiving your comments will be able to take a look at themselves and learn something about the rank situation between them. For example, if one member of the family is using the power of his voice to talk over others who have a quieter style, pointing out to him that he has many important things to say that need to be heard, but that others might like to respond in order to take the conversation further, might alert him to how dominating he is and how his loud voice is a privilege as far as being heard goes. Rather than saying to him that he is being dominant, which would result in him feeling criticized and becoming defensive, you would be framing the situation for him without blame. Why not practice a little when you notice rank discrepancy around you? Try to frame that, perhaps first mentally to yourself, and if it feels good, try saying that aloud to those involved. In doing this, you can be of great help to patients, family and staff, and also assist the unfolding of deeper and more meaningful relationships.

Having read through these chapters, you by now have a good grasp on how you can facilitate and enhance awareness in the various situations we have described, not only revealing more of the riches present for the patient, but also for the field, and for the process of death and dying. In the second part of this book we give you a variety of exercises that you may wish to try on your own, with a friend, or with the patient, in order to develop your own skills and experience in being with others at the end of life. You will be amazed at the wealth of possibilities waiting to be discovered.

Chapter 8

Conclusion

The boundaries between life and death are at best shadowy and vague. Who shall say where one ends and the other begins?

- Edgar Allen Poe

In this book and manual we have offered an array of techniques and tools that are useful in joining with others in a variety of states, supporting their process through the interventions we make, and often in helping them to complete their life journey. In presenting a process-oriented view to dementia and end of life experience, we illustrate methods and skills that provide ways in which to harness underlying dynamics, bringing deeper meaning to what is unfolding.

In Western culture we mostly find an expectation that we will live long lives. Death is something that we rarely think about or entertain. We want to be in control of our living and our dying, hoping to eradicate pain and suffering. When we are faced with death through illness, accident or aging, we go all out to preserve what we have and endeavour to get more time, sometimes using extraordinary methods, developed by medicine and technology, to achieve that.

However, in this book you will notice that the approach we use is based on an openness to the process of death and dying. Rather than push it away or ignore it, we embrace it as a guide for living. One concept that runs through each chapter in this book becomes apparent, namely, that the solution to a problem is found within the problem itself. The emphasis on digging deeper into disturbance allows us to embrace it as a potential teacher and helps us to avoid marginalizing it. In this way, we are able to welcome more of the "whole" person, enriching the person's experience through recognition of the disturber and what it holds for us. It is when we have more awareness that we become more fluid in navigating challenges and abler to avoid getting stuck in just one view or experience.

As shown throughout the book, greater inclusivity of more unknown parts enhances the journey for those with dementia, the dying, and those who accompany them. As helpers, if we can put aside our "usual" way of perceiving things, and shift to recognizing experiences that are outside of what we usually attend to, we are able to make more contact with those in far-out and altered states of consciousness. What a gift to have tools that we can use in these situations in order to support those we love and work with!

We emphasize the importance of doing our own work, being able to navigate our own unusual and altered states so that we can be with others in theirs'. The exercises offer a way to practice the skill of attending to presenting experience, as well as ways in which to notice signals and unfold them further. We also suggest cultivating an awareness of the particular attitudes or metaskills that we bring with us as we enter into interaction with those in dementia or near death. Our ability to be open, curious, loving, courageous, patient, playful and challenging can enhance experience for those with whom we interact. The development of our capacity to be *dreamlike*, not only enables us to join with the patient in their *dreamlike* experiences, but also enhances our own relationship with ourselves and our lives.

We often hear from nurses that they have little time to attend to patients' signals and even less to spend amplifying or working with them. What they have found very useful though is to make minimal interventions to support the patient's awareness. A brief intervention can be very meaningful to the patient as they feel "seen", understood and no longer alone in their inner world. The beauty of this kind of work is that the practitioner can adapt and use it according to the specific situation and experience of the person no matter what their state. Interventions can range from minimal to large movements, words and song to growls and grunts, vivid imagery to emptiness. It all rests on what is shown to us through the dreaming signals and on how we intervene and dream along with those. In addition, we also have a large range of techniques and tools that we can offer to deepen awareness and experience, depending on each unique situation.

In opening up the topic of death with our patients, their families and the staff who attend them, we are able to address the more marginalized aspects of emotional experience, support the completion of "unfinished" business, and resolve challenging relationship issues. In creating communication channels with the patient, we are able to obtain answers to questions concerning comfort and pain, and are also able to support the decision-making process for the patient and family, broaching difficult questions around life or death preferences. We can talk about how death and dying bring us face to face with our frustrations at the non-completion of certain life tasks, or about the sense of fulfilment at seeing what we have accomplished. Facing death brings an opportunity to resolve or transform perception of life tasks and to recognize the mythical journey travelled, that is now coming to an end.

In Palliative Care there is emphasis on assessing and attending to patients' and families' needs. Within the medical approach there is a need to fix and bring comfort. The process-oriented approach that we introduce in this book focuses on the experience of the patient. This is a non-pathological approach through which we discover usefulness and meaning in what is present. This book encourages us to look further than what we are used to, to support what we may usually overlook, and to unfold experience leading to greater awareness of what is trying to happen and to what may be deeply spiritual or enlightening. We hope that you find what we offer to be innovative and helpful in your interactions with patients, loved ones, and friends. We would urge you to feel free in bringing in not only what we suggest and advocate here, but also in supporting your own creativity in engaging in ways that call to you. We trust that your journeying will bring fulfilment to all concerned.

PART II

Exercises

Introduction

In this next section, we are offering you an array of exercises that you may like to practice on your own, with friends or family members, or with patients. The purpose of this section is to bring to you an opportunity for first-hand practice. In trying out these exercises you will be developing and honing skills that you will find useful in being with others. In attempting these exercises you will be learning more about, not only the methods we suggest for working with people in a range of states, but also about your own attitudes and reactions to the experiences you find both in yourself and in others, especially in the unusual states of consciousness found in dementia, delirium and during the dying process.

Our premise is that in order to support and join with others, it is necessary to know what these experiences are like from the inside out. This will better enable you to engage with them when encountered in others. In other words, being able to enter and explore unusual experiences and states of awareness within oneself, cultivates a familiarity with them as well as an understanding of how to be helpful in interacting with them when found in someone else.

We have organized these exercises by chapter to make it easier for you to read up on the theory and case studies, and then to find the accompanying exercises/s in this section of the book. As you go through them, please remember that there is no "*right*" or "*wrong*" in how you experience and unravel your own, and other's experience. The process itself, as well as the feedback you receive from those with whom you engage, will be the guides and will lead you onward as you unfold the signals and dream doors at each step, gaining insight as you go ever deeper into less known experience. The journey itself provides the riches.

Chapter 1

Death - The Transformative Process

Please be aware that your own feelings around death will influence how you approach and work with others near death or in coma. The exercise below will help to prepare you for working closely with someone near death, by noticing where your own fears and hesitations reside. It is sometimes challenging to go into an exploration, or to even imagine, your own dying process, so please pace yourself and take care of your feelings as you embark on this journey.

The Dying Experience

(You can do this exercise on your own or with a friend or partner)

• Go inside yourself and tune into your inner states. Notice your consensus reality identity and how it feels to be alive and present in the world.

• Now imagine approaching death. How do you think you will die? Will it be an accident, illness, old age or anything else? Imagine this happening. What comes up for you when anticipating dying. Take a note of your reactions and attitudes at this point and write them down or share them with your partner.

• Now slowly imagine yourself getting near to death. Experience it internally. See, hear and feel the onset. Notice the states you find yourself in as you go through this process. Take time to be in these and explore them. Notice your everyday identity dropping away as you enter the dying process.

• Notice what drops away from you in terms of how you've identified yourself, your relationship to your body, and to the world.

• As you go more and more into the dropping away and dying process notice what kinds of experiences you have here. Be mindful of the difference between your reactions to the dying process and the process itself and what it brings.

• Choose one aspect of the process and go deeply into it, entering it through image, feeling, or any way that appears to you. Become one with that experience. Take time to be in that. Notice what kind of world it evokes and how it expresses itself.

• Bring that expression into micro-movement and let your hands and then body move in that way. Take time to allow it to express itself.

• Contact the quality or essence of that movement and its nature, and give it some form of expression – perhaps a few words, poem or drawing. What is its message for you and how will you bring that into your everyday life?

Dropping Personal History

• Describe your personal history in terms of:
Gender, race, religion, profession, nationality. Your usual relationship to your body and inner state. Are you successful, popular or not. Anything about yourself you would like to mention.

• Now imagine lying dead in your grave. See all your friends and family around you, talking of all your personal qualities that are now gone.

- Allow yourself to feel all those qualities dropping away and imagine them leaving you.

- Notice what your experience is like now, freed of all of your personal history.

How do you experience that? Try to find an essential energy or core quality in that experience.

- Now imagine living from that core quality. How would you be in interaction in the world if you came from that place in yourself?

- What path would that suggest living? How could you follow that path?

- Take a few moments to imagine living in that way. Make a poem or song that integrates that.

Chapter 2

The Structure and Flow of Process

Pacing the Breath

As you do this exercise notice your own feeling responses and intuitions.

Find a friend to practice with and get them to lie down and imagine being in a coma. Ask them if there is anywhere that they would not like to be touched.

Before touching someone who is less responsive, it is important if you can, to check out if there are areas of sensitivity, pain, or if there are any trauma-related areas. Then follow the steps below.

- Let your partner know that you are with them and ask if it is okay to touch them on the wrist.

- Place your hand on your patient's wrist. Bring awareness to your touch there.

- Now pace the rhythm of their breath, pressing down gently each time they breathe in. As you talk to them try to pace this same rhythm with your voice. You may wish to hum or sing to them in that rhythm.

- Now move to another part of the body, the soles of the feet, the chest, the navel area. In each area do the same pacing of the breath while gently pressing down on the in-breath. Notice any tiny reactions that your partner may have.

- Notice your own reactions and feelings as you approach your partner and touch them. Are you shy, excited, cautious, brusque, unfeeling, repelled, frightened, etc. What is your style of touching and what metaskills (feeling attitudes) do you recognize?

- Watch for feedback.

- Give feedback to your partner about what was helpful.

You can also try this out placing your hands on the soles of your partner's feet. Once you've had some practice with this, you may also want to try it out on a patient, or loved one in an altered state of near death.

• Let your partner know that you are with them and ask if it is okay to touch them on the wrist.

• Place your hand on your patient's wrist. Bring awareness to your touch there.

• Now pace the rhythm of their breath, pressing down gently each time they breathe in. As you talk to them try to pace this same rhythm with your voice.

• Notice tiny signals that appear and comment on them, bringing awareness to them. Relate to these signals, metacommunicating about them.

• Now choose one signal and begin to amplify it. Be creative in intervening with it, trying some of the ways we have discussed. Watch for feedback.

• Continue to interact with this signal until there is either a shift or loss of energy. Now choose another signal and try the same as above.

• Give your partner time to come out of his/her state and when ready get feedback about the interventions made and metaskills used.

Once you've had some practice with this, you may also want to try it out on a patient, or loved one in an altered state or near death.

Amplification

Best to practice this with a friend or family member. You can also practice by yourself or with a patient or loved one.

• Sit with your partner, say hello, chat to them, pace the breath through touch, and watch for feedback.

• Notice the signals present in the patient such as a blink, movement of finger or foot or other part of body, raising an eyebrow, puckering lips.

• Choose one signal and focus on it. Bring awareness to that signal by describing it verbally to the patient, connecting with it through touch, and amplifying it for them. Watch for feedback.

• Take time to experiment with amplifying it. Be creative in the ways you do this. You can metacommunicate about what you notice; use light touch or vibration; movement; make a sound, rhythm or tune to go along with the signal; create a story about it; or draw it if the patient is able to do that. Help the patient with his/her awareness by metacommunicating about what you notice.

• If you feel ready to move on, choose another signal and repeat steps 3 and 4.

• Give your partner time to come out of their state. Get feedback from them on what worked for them, your interventions and style.

Choose a friend or family member to be your partner.

• The person who is doing the work (A = friend/family member) will stand in their usual posture and you as the practitioner (B) will take time to walk around A and observe him/her.

• As B, do you notice anything about A's posture that doesn't quite fit in with the rest of their body position, or that in some way appears out of alignment.

• Using a minimal intervention, and with the permission of A, make a slight adjustment to A's posture.

• Now A, notice what it is like for you as you adopt this new posture. Notice how you feel, what happens to your image of yourself, and what your attitude to the world is like in this position. What kind of quality, or way of being is evoked by this new posture?

• Experiment going back and forth between your original posture and the new one. What does the original position evoke for you in terms of feeling, image of yourself, and attitude to life and how does this change with the new position.

• Give voice to this way of being evoked by the new posture. Allow it to speak, sing or make up a poem that best expresses itself. Give it a name.

• If you like, you may switch positions with your friend/family member so that you also get a chance to be the subject.

Chapter 3

Far-Out and Altered States of Consciousness

The exercises below will familiarize you with a range of states of consciousness and provide you with a degree of fluidity in navigating out-of-ordinary states, both in yourself and others.

Working with your own Altered State

- Think about your life at present and a question you may have about it, or about yourself. Write that down and put it aside.
- Make yourself comfortable. Bring your attention onto yourself and your body.

- Use your attention to scan your feelings and body experiences, and notice what is present for you. Notice what it is like for you to go inside and bring awareness to your inner states.

- Now remember a time when you were in an altered state. Bring that state into the moment and allow yourself to enter it now. Notice what that is like for you. What are the feelings you experience, your body states, what catches your attention?

- Staying with the state and the experience of "dreaminess", make up a story about yourself and your experience of being altered. Keep going with the story until it comes to a natural conclusion or something shifts for you.

- Slowly coming out of the state, ask yourself how does this story reflect on your question from 1, if at all. Does it have a message for you in your everyday life?

Dreaming and Intuiting

(Both Partners can do this together at the same time.)

- Sit with your partner without verbal communication.

- Allow yourself to gaze at them and at the same time enter a slightly dreamy state of awareness.

• Now begin to intuit and dream about them while gazing at them, letting their appearance, e.g. colours, shapes, sizes, and their signals speak to you.

• Form a dream-like image of who they are and what their inner/outer life might be like.

• Share with partner and check in with them about how close your dreaming might be to their experience of themselves.

Binary Communication[39]

This exercise can be tried with a patient in an altered state, coma or close to death. You may also wish to try first with a friend in order to get feedback from them about the usefulness of your interventions.

• Sit with a partner and take a few moments to notice and pace the breathing. Tell the person you are there. Press the wrist on the inhalation.

• Notice any signals – a slight movement of the finger or mouth, raising of an eyebrow, a twitch of the foot, turning of the head, a slight sound or another signal.

---

[39] Mindell, Amy (1999). *Coma: A healing journey*

- Establish communication with this signal by commenting about it. *"I notice your finger moving. You can use that finger to communicate"* Place your hands slightly on the area where the signal originates to give the person more access to that particular signal. Wait for feedback. Each time the signal occurs remark excitedly about it, and encourage the use of the signal to communicate. Example: If noticing a slight movement on the person's chin, place your hands gently on the chin to increase the person's awareness of that to make the signal more accessible to them. For a sound, you can make this sound and put your hands on the person's lips or gently on the throat; alternatively, you could place their hand on your lips or throat. Tell them that they can use that signal to communicate with if they choose. Then wait and see if there is a response.

- After trying that a number of times, if there is no response, try another signal. Repeat the above.

- Once you have established a signal of communication, you can set up a binary system. Tell the person that when s/he makes that particular signal or movement it will mean, "yes" as for example, "you can use that signal to communicate. If you want to say "yea" then raise your eyebrow. If you want to say no, you needn't do anything".

- Ask if this system is OK and watch for a response. If "yes" then you can begin to ask questions. Tell the person that in a moment you will ask them some questions. Give him time to prepare inwardly. Then speaking slowly ask the person a yes or no question, such as, "are you in pain"? Notice any responses.

- Do you want to come out? Do you want to remain in that state? Do you want to die? Do you want to go on living? If unsure of the answers wait and then ask again – another day.

• Experiment with your partner and when you feel complete bring the exercise to an end and get feedback from your partner as to what was useful and what not so useful.

Chapter 4

Whose Reality is this Anyway?

Exploring Delirium

- Focus on your breath for a few moments

- Remember a time when you experienced some delirium or someone you know did or imagine what it might be like.

- Go into a cloudy, foggy, delirium state – just a little bit.

- Look at yourself with an inner eye (meta-communicator) from that state. What do you see? What sounds do you hear – inside and outside? Make a sound that goes with this.

- Keep going and feel into the state and make a movement that goes along with it – sensing into it.

- Now pick up the sound and movement and amplify them while noticing your experiences. Take some time with this.

- As you amplify, notice who makes that sound and moves this way. What figure is there? – a scared one? wild one? ecstatic one? angry one? It could be a mythical figure or animal.

- Go further with your experience adding gestures, facial expressions, movements and postures. As you do that, feel its quality or essence. You can do that by slowing it down or feeling into its beginnings. Find a place in nature that has this quality or energy.

- Be in that place – feel into it, be it, make a hand movement that matches the energy of that place. Take a few moments to be there.

- Ask how its energy can help you with the delirium state you started out with. The answer may come non-verbally, as a feeling, a picture or movement.

- Also ask how this energy or presence could help you with others experiencing delirium, family members, staff.

- How might the world view you if you were to embody this more?

- Make a few notes and then share.

Discovering the Magic in Forgetfulness: Exploring Dementia

(Optimal if you can do this exercise with someone else who can keep a record for you)

• With your partner talk about your own experiences of forgetfulness, if any.

• Imagine a time in the future when you may develop Alzheimer's/dementia. Imagine yourself then. How do you look? How do you talk or make noise? Feel how your body would feel, notice the posture you would be in, move as you imagine yourself moving then, and breathe how you would breathe. Take your time to act this out.

• As you act that out, be there in that Alzheimer's/dementia state and notice your attitude to life. Describe it to your partner who will write it down for you.

• Go further into this state and notice what it is like to leave all that was known behind you. What new state does this bring for you?

• What would it be like to integrate more of this state into your everyday life? Where and how might it be helpful?

- Bring to mind a patient or someone you know who suffers from dementia.
- Imagine being them and then actually become them in your feelings, body experiences, postures, sounds and verbal expression, and style of relating.
- Your partner engages and interacts with you as the patient using channel experiences, mirroring, going further, dreaming into the patient's experience, following feedback and helping to complete the process.
- Practitioner to watch for your own edges and try to cross them.
- Chat together and find out what was useful and give general feedback.

Chapter 5

Metaphor, Dreams and Spirituality

Diving into Essence

• Take a few moments to find a comfortable position, close your eyes and allow your awareness to become cloudy.

• Take some time there, letting go of your usual way of attending.

• Remaining clouded, allow your eyes to open minimally and move your gaze around the room until something catches your attention. Notice what exactly about that pulls your attention.

• Now imagine a whole realm of just that quality – it may be a colour, shape, texture, size, etc. Allow yourself to enter that realm and merge with it. Notice what the atmosphere, energy and quality of that world is like. Go into the deepest essence of that and allow yourself to be there.

•   Try to keep awareness and notice what subtle tendency or sentient-like experience exists there. Let yourself become that.

•   Now begin to move spontaneously, hum or make a sound that is generated by that experience. Keep going with that … perhaps a poem, song or dance emerges.

•   Does that have any meaning for you and for your everyday self, and if so, what?

Discovering the Dreaming behind a Dream Figure or Symbol

•   Think of a recent dream or dream-like experience which has made an impact on you.

•   Notice the dream figures or symbols in the dream. Pick one and describe it with as much detail as possible. Explore this dream figure/symbol by talking about it, drawing it.

•   Notice if there is anything forbidden or forgotten about this. What story or memory does it evoke in you?

•   Now imagine being that dream figure/symbol. Feel your way into it and notice how it feels. Make a movement that expresses that feeling. Add sound or words. Keep going until you discover its essential nature.

• What quality, essence or energy does it hold within it. Feel this essence and let it unfold by giving you a message or guidance about a course of action. What advice does this have for you?

• Imagine bringing this quality or essence and its message into everyday life.

Process Mind and Dreaming[40]

• Think of a situation or difficulty that is challenging to you. Where or how might you get stopped in addressing this in the way you would like? Write it down and put it aside.

• Now, stand and sense your deepest self, whatever that means to you in the moment and ask yourself where you sense that deepest self in your body. When you have found it, use your breath to amplify the feeling in that part of your body. Breathe into it and let a motion and a sound arise from that part of your body.

• When you are ready, associate a spot or a place on earth that most closely corresponds to that feeling. Choose a spot and go there in your imagination.

---

[40] Exercise from workshop with Arny and Amy Mindell

• Imagine standing, sitting, or lying in that spot. Sense its atmosphere and its presence. Let it dream its way into you. Let it move you and make sounds or songs through you.

• Become this spot. From the point of view of this spot, look back at your ordinary self and give yourself some tips or advice.

• How might the quality of your earthspot, and its advice, be useful to the situation named above. Imagine bringing that into the situation and notice the effect it has.

• Does this experience remind you of anything you have been exploring in your dreams/self-exploration/spiritual work?

Inner Work on Communication Style41

• Think of a difficulty or conflict that you are facing or have faced. This can be with a friend, family member, patient, or colleague.

• Think of your usual style when addressing this difficulty– what is your mood like, your posture, attitude, tone of voice, movements, etc.

• Put all of this aside.

---

41 Thanks to Amy Mindell for this exercise

- Now make a squiggle on your paper. Look at it and notice part of the squiggle that stands out for you.

- Take the part that stands out and draw it on its own.

- Now bring that drawing into movement and sound.

- What kind of style does that evoke for you?

- What would that style be like in terms of mood, attitude, posture, tone of voice, etc., and what would its expression and energy be like.

- Try that now.

- Where and how would that more secondary style be useful for you in your difficulty in the first part of the exercise and in life-in general?

Chapter 6

Pain – The Ultimate Disturber

Working with the Pain Maker

- Take a moment to check in with your body and choose a pain to focus on.
- Place your attention on the feeling of the pain and the sensations that are present there. Describe the pain in detail using sensory-grounded information. Try not to focus on the effects of the pain but on the experience of the pain itself and the sensations there. For example, if you have a headache which is throbbing and makes you feel frustrated, don't focus on the frustration but on the energy within the experience of throbbing.
- Now, as you feel this pain, go ahead and amplify it as if you were creating this pain on someone else. You might use a cushion or something else handy that will facilitate you doing this. If it is a pressure or tightness, for example, create that on your cushion, stuffed animal, or whatever is handy.

- Go right into becoming the pain maker – feel and move like it, take on its posture, voice, and facial expression. Keep amplifying and playing this out until you get a sense of the character who creates this pain and what motivates it. You might also get an insight into its quality and nature.

- Is there anything useful in this figure for you? Where does this live in you and how might you marginalize it.

- Imagine using this quality on a daily basis. How and where will it be useful?

Personifying Pain[42].

(You might choose to do this exercise with a partner, or you can also try it on your own)

- Take some time to check in with your body to see if you are experiencing any pain in the moment. There may be a couple of places – choose one. If there is currently no pain you might have a memory of a particular pain you experienced at some point, or a pain that you dread having. It might also be pain that you observed somebody else experiencing, like a patient or loved one.

---

[42] This exercise sparked by a practice from Lama Tsultrim – *Feeding your Demons*

158

- Imagine having that pain now. Locate where you hold it most strongly in your body and intensify the sensation. Become aware of the qualities of the sensation in your body and describe them to your partner in detail, or write them down. Use sensory grounded descriptions, e.g. it is sharp, dull, hot, cold, piercing, pressure, throbbing, comes and goes, etc.

- Now personify this sensation as a figure with arms, legs, eyes, or it could be a force of nature or an animate being. Notice its character, emotional state, size, the way it moves, looks at you. What motivates it? What does it want? Name that and share with your partner.

- Now imagine giving that figure what it wants. Your partner could play out the figure. Keep feeding it what it desires – feel free to switch roles back and forth with your partner as you go further with the interaction.

- Notice if anything shifts both in your experience and in the figure. Does it begin to transform in any way, and if so, how? Do you also transform?

- How would this shift inform you as you deal with your experience of pain and its effects?

Unfolding Pain to find an Ally

- Take some time to check in with your body to see if you are experiencing any pain in the moment. There may be a couple of places – choose one. If there is currently no pain you might have a memory of a particular pain you experienced at some point, or a pain that you dread having. It might also be pain that you observed somebody else experiencing, like a patient or loved one.

• Imagine having that pain now. Locate where you hold it most strongly in your body and intensify the sensation. Become aware of the qualities of the sensation in your body and describe them to your partner in detail, or write them down. Use sensory grounded descriptions, e.g. it is sharp, dull, hot, cold, piercing, pressure, throbbing, comes and goes, etc.

• In proprioception, amplify the quality of the pain that stands out most for you. Keep going with it until the channel shifts and an image or sound arises. Keep amplifying this new experience until you get a sense of the style of being that this image or sound evokes. Bring in some movement if you can. How does this figure or style operate – what is its core nature like? Would this be useful for you to integrate too?

• Now go further and discover the essence of the pain. Begin by making the sound softer and moving less and less while feeling the same energy until you find its subtlest tendency. Keep expressing this tendency until you find its essence – its pre-verbal, pre-manifest, form. Allow yourself to fill up with this essence. Take some moments with it.

• When ready ask yourself: How might everyday life be different if I were to live this essence more? Is there a glimpse of it already present there? What do I need to do to support myself to bring this in more?

• Make some notes and/or share with a friend.

Chapter 7

Relationships, Families, Systems

Exploring a Relationship Disturber

• Think of a person who you find disturbing in some way. What is it about them that irritates, upsets or disturbs you? Describe it to yourself and/or make a few notes. If you like, you can even make a quick sketch of that person or the disturbing feature.

• Now, almost as if putting yourself aside, step into being the other – that disturbing person. Move and make gestures like they do, take on their posture, voice, speech pattern, their inner feelings and motivations. Allow yourself to step into your dream of how they are, both in their expressions and in their inner worlds.

• Keep going with that experience until some deep insight into their nature occurs and you get an "aha" flash of how they function and what motivates them.

• Remaining in the experience of being that other, imagine looking at yourself across the room. Looking through this other's eyes, what do you notice about yourself – what stands out that you have not been aware of before?

• Make a few notes both about what you have discovered about the other, and also about yourself. Does this change your perspective of the relationship in any way, and if so how?

• Now that you have more insight about both of you, how is this a learning for you? What does the disturbance bring you that wakes you up in some way? How could this be helpful?

• Imagine interacting with the person from this place. The next time you are with them try bringing in your new insight and learning.

The Space Between People

Sit with someone and chat, or if you know the person discuss some challenge that might exist between you in your relationship.

Part A - on your own:

• Become quiet and notice the atmosphere between you two now in the moment or at the time of the difficulty. What is the quality, colour, or sound?

Imagine a landscape or weather system that could represent it. What are the movement tendencies in that landscape or weather system?

• Take a paper and pen. Sketch the landscape or weather system. Take the most intense, disturbing or intriguing element of your picture and on another sheet of paper draw a picture expressing that element and give it a name.

• Hold it in front of your face. As you do so, notice the movements that arise in your body and follow them a little, feeling into this element.

Part B – with your partner:

• Share your experience with your partner. How are your experiences similar or different? What interactional style would your drawing suggest (for example passionate, quiet, poetic, dry, direct, hinting at things and so forth)?

• Go back to interacting. Experiment with including the viewpoints and styles of your landscape or weather system. Speak to the other from that place. Use it as a quality and feeling skill in interaction and explore.

• What learning or inspiration comes to you through this interaction? Think of a way to express this more in your relationships generally and in the world.

Working with Moods
High/Low Dreaming in Relationship

• Think of a relationship in which you experience some challenge or difficulty. Describe that relationship a little to your partner or to yourself if you are working alone.

• What is your high dream for that relationship? In other words, what is your highest hope, vision or longing of how that relationship could be? Describe that to your partner or yourself.

• Imagine that the relationship is that way. Go into the state that the high dream would bring you and give it expression through gesture, posture, voice, movement, a poem. Make a quick energy sketch of that.

• Now, think of what happens when that is not achieved in the relationship. What kind of mood do you get into? Describe that to your partner or to yourself.

• Go into that state – the low dream experience – and give it expression through gesture, posture, voice, movement, a poem. Make a quick energy sketch of that.

• Go back and forth now between the high and low dream state, acting each out and creating a dance between the two. Keep going until some shift, insight or resolution happens. What way of being or energy does the shift bring you? Make a third energy sketch of that.

• How would this quality be helpful in the challenging or difficult relationship described in (1)?

• Discuss with your partner or make some notes for yourself.

You can do this exercise with a friend or family member. Do part A on your own and then come together with your exercise partner to complete part B.

Part A – Inner Work

Take some time on your own to think about:

• Where you feel privileged in your life. Is that in terms of age, gender, education level, physical condition, ethnic group, relationship status, spiritual background...etc?

• How do you perceive yourself acting from this position of rank? Do you pick it up easily, feel comfortable with it, or does it tend to be more marginalized or hidden?

• Take on your privileges, feel your rank in the above areas now and notice your experience. How is your posture, movement, speech, tone of voice and how do you feel about yourself? Act this out a little.

• Now think about where you feel less privileged. Is that in terms of age, gender, education level, physical condition, ethnic group, relationship status, spiritual background ... etc? How do you react to this perception? How might it influence your interaction with others?

• Notice your experience when you identify with having less privilege. How is your posture, movement, speech, tone of voice and how do you feel about yourself? Act this out a little.

•   Which part is more familiar to you and more integrated, and which do you think is more marginalized and needs more support?

Part B —Come together with your partner.

Both to do this piece at the same time.

•   Go ahead now in your interaction with your partner and support the more marginalized part by amplifying it and bringing it out more fully. Express it in the relationship channel with your partner and have a relationship interaction together bringing in this lesser-known part.

•   What does this bring for yourself and for the relationship that is useful to you personally and to your friendship and ongoing interaction?

•   Share together about ways to support this in your lives and what you learned about your own rank from this exercise.

The Wounded Healer and Deepest Gifts of the Facilitator

•   Think of a troublesome or disturbing scene you've encountered where you felt triggered and unable to maintain your usual awareness.

- What was problematic for you in that situation with yourself or others? Describe/remember that experience and all the feeling reactions that went along with it. Make a small hand movement to express that difficulty.

- Imagine being very old and wise and that you have done many great things in your life and for the people around you. You feel fulfilled by your life. Take a moment and allow yourself to experience that fullness. Make a small hand movement with your other hand to express this state of being.

- Give time for both hands to move their experience and notice how they meet, influence or interact with each other. Give that space and take time with that. Allow the hands to come to a momentary resolution.

- What new feeling attitude or skill emerges from the meeting of your hands? Name it and write a poem/song or do a drawing of it.

- What approach might it suggest for the disturbance you experience in (1)? What does it offer you for your further work with relationships and groups?

7. How might this also be useful in your ongoing work and also other areas of your life?

Analysis of a Field: Practice

- Bring to mind a particular field, context or environment in which you are engaged with others, or have been in the past, where you feel challenged or where the atmosphere is difficult to negotiate.
- Think of that field situation, the people involved and the dynamics present.
- What roles exist in that field? As you think about that, begin to name the roles and write them down, or place each role within a circle you have drawn, giving them a spot in that circle.
- Continue naming the roles and placing them in the circle and as you do so notice which roles are polarized against each other and which seem to be more in sync with each other.
- Now think about the ghost roles that may be present – those energies, belief systems or figures that influence the field, but that may not be so apparent. Place them also in the circle.
- Take some time now to practice metacommunicating about what you notice in the field in terms of atmosphere, how the roles interact with each other, and the underlying feelings that may be present. Give yourself time to find the phrases or descriptions that seem to fit best and that may be helpful to the field. If you like you can even imagine being one or more of the roles and try out how the metacommunication may be received by each role.

- When you feel complete, ask yourself what you've learned from this exercise and how this can be useful when you next find yourself in a challenging field. What was particularly useful that you would like to remember to use again. Write that down.

REFERENCES

Alexander, E. (2012). *Proof of Heaven: A Neurosurgeon's Journey into the Afterlife*. New York: Simon and Schuster.

Bandler, R. & Grinder, J. (1979). *Frogs into Princes: The Introduction to Neuro-Linguistic Programming*. California: Real People Press.

Betty, L. Stafford (2006). Are they Hallucinations or are they Real? The Spirituality of Deathbed and Near-Death Visions. *Omega Journal of Death and Dying 53, 37-49.*

Bulkeley, K. & Bulkley, P. (2005). *Dreaming Beyond Death: A Guide to Pre-Death Dreams and Visions*. Boston: Beacon Press.

Castaneda, C. (1981). *The Eagle's Gift*. London: Penguin Group

Gutkind, L. (ed.) (2011). *Twelve Breaths a Minute: End-of-Life Essays*. Dallas: Southern Methodist University Press.

Jenkinson, S. (2015). *Die Wise: A Manifesto of Sanity and Soul.* California: North Atlantic Books.

Iordache, S. (2012). Palliative People's Dreams and Dream Related Perceptions and Interpretations. A mixed method investigation. Thesis in partial fulfilment for Degree of Doctor of Philosophy in Psychology. New Zealand: Auckland University.

Lakoff, G. & Johnson, M. (1980). *Metaphors We Live By.* Illinois: University of Chicago Press.

Levine, S. & Levine, O. (1982). *Who Dies?* New York: Doubleday.

Lewin, K. (1943). Defining the "Field at a Given Time". *Psychological Review 50: 292-310.*

Mindell, Amy. (1994/2001). *Metaskills: the Spiritual Art of Therapy.* Portland, Oregon: Lao Tse Press.

Mindell, Amy. (1999). *Coma: A healing Journey. A Guide for Family, Friends, and Helpers.* Portland, Oregon: Lao Tse Press.

Mindell, Arnold. (1984). *Working with the Dreaming Body.* London: Penguin-Arkana.

Mindell, Arnold. (1992). *The Leader as Martial Artist.* San Francisco: Harper.

Mindell, Arnold. (1995). *Sitting in the Fire*. Portland, Oregon: Lao Tse Press.

Mindell, Arnold. (2008). *Coma. The Dreambody near Death*. Portland, Oregon: Lao Tse Press.

Morin, P. (2015). *Health in Sickness, Sickness in Health. Toward a New Process-oriented Medicine*. Oregon: Deep Democracy Exchange.

Morin, P. & Reiss, G. (2010). *Inside Coma: A New View of Awareness, Healing, and Hope*. USA: Praeger.

Parnia, S. (2013). *Erasing Death*. New York: HarperCollins.

Richards, T. & Tomandl, S. (2006). *An Alzheimer's surprise party: New sentient Communication Skills and Insights for Understanding and Relating to People with Dementia*. Illinois: Lulu Press Inc.

Sacks, O. (2012). *Hallucinations*. New York: Random House.

Scott, L. (2014). Out of the Matrix. Unpublished manuscript in partial fulfilment of Diploma in Process Work, ANZPOP.

Shabahangi, N. & Szymkiewicz, B. (2008). *Deeper into Soul: Beyond Dementia and Alzheimer's toward Forgetfulness Care.* San Francisco: Elders Academy Press.

Storr, A. (1983). *The Essential Jung: Selected Writings.* New Jersey: Princeton University Press.

von Franz, M-L. (1984) (trans. Kennedy, E.X. & Brooks, V.) *On Dreams and Death: A Jungian interpretation.* Boston: Shambhala Inc.